SORRY
for your
LOSS

SORRY
for your
LOSS

What working with the
dead taught me about *life*

KATE MARSHALL
with LINDA WATSON-BROWN

MARDLE

First published in 2022 by Mardle Books
15 Church Road
London, SW13 9HE
www.mardlebooks.com

Text © 2022 Kate Marshall

Paperback ISBN 9781914451560
eBook ISBN 9781914451690

A CIP catalogue record for this book is available from the British Library.

Every reasonable effort has been made to trace copyright-holders of material
reproduced in this book, but if any have been inadvertently overlooked the
publishers would be glad to hear from them.

Printed in the UK

10 9 8 7 6 5 4 3 2 1

Cover image: Arcangel

This book is dedicated to everyone who has lost
someone, particularly those who were denied
the chance to say goodbye.

And as always, to my amazing family.

Love you all bibbies.

xxxxx

Whilst all of the stories within this memoir are true, names have been changed as have some of the background details. We all deserve respect – and that shouldn't stop when we are dead.

Before
Early 2019

I didn't start with the dead. I started with hoarders.

"What do you think I should expect?"

"Well now, let's see... houses that are death traps due to the sheer quantity of accumulated rubbish. Rooms that are crammed from floor to ceiling with enough orders from QVC to keep them going for decades. People lying in their own filth, surrounded by takeaway boxes, who couldn't find a path to the kitchen if their lives depended on it. More animal faeces than you'd see in a zoo. That sort of thing. Here you go."

With those words from my new boss, Gina, I was handed an industrial boilersuit, a mask and thick gloves. This was my job now. I was going to help people who hoarded, encourage them to clear their houses, and hopefully change their lives.

I learned very quickly that the clients don't think you're there because they're living in squalor – they don't think they're hoarding in the first place, so most don't identify as hoarders. They think that any help they are given is for something small; maybe a pile of boxes they can't manage to move that is a health hazard, or perhaps the dishes need doing (the ones that have been sitting there for three years). There was hardly ever an acknowledgment that their compulsion was completely out of hand. It was always just a "few" things, a "bit" of a muddle. There were always excuses, too. The bins only got emptied twice a month and the neighbours filled them up anyway. Everything would get used at some point or someone else might need it. The company might stop making it or it might run out.

Within my first few weeks, I felt like I'd heard it all. One man had his wall recesses lined with empty wine bottles.

"What's with that then, Colin?" I asked.

"My collection?" he asked, smiling with pride. "A lot of them are very rare, you know. They're worth a lot of money, so you be careful. They'll be worth a fortune one day."

I looked at his "collection" of hundreds of dusty Skol lager and Blue Nun empties… and wondered how to break the news. Then realised there was no news to break, as Colin wouldn't be getting rid of these in a hurry.

Clients would consistently tell me that they had no time to make a start on things, even though they were in bed all day and most never left the house.

"Where do you keep the binbags?" I'd ask breezily. "I just need to pop a few things out."

"No point in buying them, love." I'd be told. "You ever tried to open one of those buggers?"

Cat litter trays quickly became my nemesis. I've got a strong stomach, but every time I saw one brimming over, maggots wriggling, I'd heave. There was rarely just one. Instead, there would be a few as, rather than empty and clean what was there, they tended to get another – but never throw the old one out. They'd be teeming with white crawling things, like some horrific science experiment in the kitchen.

"I don't think I can face another cat litter tray," I told Gina. "Anyone with a non-maggot issue by any chance?"

She flicked through her files wearily. "Where to start, where to start… Ah, here we go. Lena. She's lovely. I did her assessment. Really nice old lady – and no cats."

Lena was indeed lovely, and at least everything was in a box. Everything. I squeezed down the hallway with boxes on either side, into the spare room which had about 40 kettles, more toasters, and even more George Foreman grills.

"You've got a lot of kettles there, Lena," I mentioned, as if it was just a passing comment.

"Just in case, love, just in case," she told me, with an extremely serious expression.

"What's the story there, then?" There was always a story.

"You won't believe this, but can you imagine there was one time when my kettle broke – and on the very same day, so did my friend Hetty's! What a day that was, what a day. I'll never be in a pickle like that again. Now, if that ever happens to you, love, you know where to come."

"And the grills? What about them?"

"I always say, you just can't beat a George Foreman grill. They come in a lot of different types, you know."

I knew now! "What about we sell a few of these? Make you a bit of cash? That would be good wouldn't it?"

Lena looked at me warily. "How many were you thinking of?"

"Maybe we could keep one and sell the rest?"

I didn't know until that day, just how many different George Foreman grills existed in the world. We couldn't sell that one because it was a two-slice. We couldn't sell that one because it was a four-slice. We couldn't sell that one because it was non-stick. We couldn't sell that one because it was a nice box. We couldn't sell that one because Lena had heard it was very hard to come by.

We couldn't sell any of them. A bit of shifting about and Lena was sure we'd done a grand job.

"How about a cup of tea to celebrate?" she asked. Well, we wouldn't be short of a kettle...

Of course, it wasn't about toasters or grills, it was about loss and not wanting to let go. It was about keeping some tiny sliver of control in a world that was becoming increasingly scary for an old woman like Lena. Genuine hoarders had tangible items; it wasn't about cleaning, as some of them actually had spotless houses. They just couldn't move for stuff. It was this stuff which gave them more comfort than the need to be able to move around their own house. They often had trauma in their background but their circumstances were different to the clients whose homes were filthy, the people who had never really cleaned. The years of lying in their own muck just accumulated. These clients had generally given up on life; there would often be alcohol and drug issues, relationships had broken down and there were no family or friends in the picture. They saw no-one from one day until the next. I found that these were usually younger people and there was a pattern of simply not moving from the couch or bed, unless it was to get food or alcohol.

One man had hundreds of plastic milk bottles filled with urine. He lay on his bed, day after day – a bed that wasn't fit for a dog – just watching TV, smoking, and not even bothering to get up for the loo. Judging by the smell of the house, there were the results of other bodily functions being left about the place as well. He was completely desensitised to how disgusting it was; the smell of cat urine which made my eyes sting, the curtain of flies which hung over everything. He'd previously been "given assistance" and cleaned out three times. Skips had been brought in and, as usually happens, once it's all cleared, everything underneath is ruined. He'd been given new floors, new furniture, and the whole house had been painted – but no help was given to break the cycle. It was uninhabitable again within 12 months and the whole process would start all over again as soon as I left.

That's not OK.

I quickly realised that these people needed support, they needed help and the real things in life – a reason to get up in the morning and a sense of self-worth – not a debit card with auto-fill details for every website.

It's so easy to get things online now, with shopping channels available every minute of every day. All the overseas-selling websites – the cheapandandnasty.com brigade – are a dream come true for people who have little to look forward to in life, other than the arrival of tat from China that appears as if by magic. The addiction of getting deliveries, the rush that comes when they hear the van or the postie, gives them something they might not be getting from anything else. Clients would tell me that they hadn't gone looking for things, bargains had just "popped" up and they couldn't resist. Some of them started Christmas shopping in January, buying as much stuff in sales as they could without ever really knowing who it was for. Constant sales in the shops and online stores facilitate this sort of behaviour, as there is always some great reduction on something to be had, never mind if it's needed or not.

It's gradual, you don't wake up one day with a house like that. There were times when, doing big clean ups, I'd find envelopes filled with cash and ten-pound notes under the sofa, yet no-one in the house was eating that night. Other people would say they were too skint to buy a bottle of kitchen cleaner but they'd order takeaways every night. It was almost as if they'd disconnected from the true value of things and life was just a meaningless search for instant, fleeting pleasures.

I did enjoy helping people and I did become immune to most of the sights and smells after just a few weeks, but there was such frustration with the sticking plaster approach. I knew that my work was just a temporary fix that wasn't addressing the real problem. Sometimes, I could even see rooms filling up while I was there – I'd sort one room, move onto the next, with the client behind me "rescuing" some of the discarded rubbish quicker than I could get rid of it.

One woman had piles of newspapers floor to ceiling, filling one entire room. I now know that you can get 4000 in one pile. They were all vitally important apparently, every single one; but they were never looked at and the bugs teeming out in all directions meant that they would disintegrate as soon as they were moved, anyway. This type of hoarder tended to be older women, while it was men in the 20-50 age group who were the hardest to help. They would fall into the dirty category rather than the hoarding one – and what they hoarded was mess. Almost without exception they would be drinkers, smokers, or drug users. They'd generally have no social circle and say that they had no need to engage with anybody. They often used pornography all day, every day, and had lost all connection with the real world. Bottles, cans, cigarette butts would all pile up around them and they couldn't care less. With some people – almost always women – I could see there was a fluid line between personal possessions and junk, but this was different.

Even with filthy houses, the ones I'd been warned about, I'd never go straight in with my boilersuit and gloves on. These were people who needed to make a connection and there wouldn't be a chance of any progress if they thought I was judging them from the first visit. Of course, some people couldn't be helped, some wouldn't even answer me, but the ones who gave me a glimmer of hope made it worthwhile.

"Let's make tiny, baby steps," I'd suggest. "Next time, I'll wear protective clothing just to make sure all your precious things don't come to harm." That would give me a reason to come in my full garb without making them feel awful.

At the start, I genuinely thought I could make a difference. I thought a clean room would stay a clean room but 99.9 per cent of the clients would never – *could* never for many of them – change. The rule was that none of us was allowed to throw anything away unless the person had explicitly agreed to it going. It was like negotiating a UN treaty. I'd sit with them for three or four hours and they'd accept me throwing out the dirty cotton buds on the floor. One woman kept her baby in a highchair all day as there was a sea of rubbish underneath, but she only allowed me to pick up some filthy tissues. I'd suggest filling a box with things for a car boot sale, as many of them claimed that was why they were saving things. But, at the end of it, there would be no more than a couple of bits of cardboard and some flyers put aside. It was so slow, like plaiting sawdust.

There's no denying that there was a huge amount of frustration with the job but, when there was satisfaction, it was heart-warming. One woman had lost her son. Martha had been his carer and she'd lived off toasties when he was alive, as there was no time to make meals for herself. When he died, she hoarded toastie and panini machines. I couldn't see the floor for them, I couldn't even see a chair. People often accumulate medication and Martha had six bottles of morphine down the side of the sofa – just in case. That was a phrase I heard so often and it was a safety net, really. *Just in case, just in case.*

It took four weeks of visits and talking but, she ended up engaging so well, we cleared the whole ground floor. I really did feel that Martha would stick to what we planned and build on what had been achieved. But what she needed more than anything was bereavement counselling and support. Without her son, she had nothing, she had no purpose – and tidying up wasn't going to solve that.

People weren't living their lives and I felt the only difference I could make was being a presence, talking to them, but it was a box-ticking exercise for the housing authority. There was no joined-up thinking at all between services. There was also no distinction made between hoarding urine or hoarding toasters. But there is, there's a huge difference. Some people would move on to have a life if they were given what they were crying out for, some people would rather live in their own filth no matter what was offered. It was a temporary fix without putting support in place. I could walk away but they were still sat in filth.

They'd given up on themselves and their environment – a nice life was something for other people So many people hadn't even used their own bathroom in years.

The number of people who used carrier bags instead of the toilet was unbelievable. Other people would have their cooker or toilet or fridge full of other things – shoes, power tools, collectibles. One lady had done beautiful crafting thirty years ago – cards and crochet, embroidery in frames. She'd become a widow at a young age, never crafted again, but continued to buy everything for crafting, filling rooms from floor to ceiling. The bathroom was piled high with die cutting machines, each of them worth hundreds of pounds; it looked like a warehouse in there. She had "one day" syndrome as so many clients did – one day she'd get back to it, one day she'd use everything.

I started thinking about these people and their lives all the time. I felt guilty if I enjoyed myself. I sat in my completely uncluttered house after a day's work and thought that I didn't deserve it. Why did some people draw the short straw in life? I thought about it constantly, the worry was relentless and I was exhausted.

One day, it just became too much. Sent to a client called Clive, I walked in and it felt like Groundhog Day. Piles of newspapers in the hallway. Half-eaten pizza boxes lying on every surface. The usual bottles filled with yellow liquid. The all-too-common stench of something that I knew needed to be in the toilet rather than down the back of the sofa where Clive lay, immobile and immersed in something vile on his phone.

I looked around me at the chaos and despair. *This is no way to live*, I thought.

And I wasn't just talking about Clive.

Something had to change. My life had to change. I had to discover what mattered and where I could make a difference.

Chapter 1
May 2019

L ife wasn't being lived by so many and I was massively disillusioned by the lack of support. If support had been in place in any effective way, lots of these people could have had their worlds completely changed. I'd always wanted to help people with their mental state (my previous job had been in mental health – again, there was very little support), and I knew that would have to be at the heart of any new role I took on. An inordinate amount of people never get over loss and I had a feeling that was the key to whatever move I'd make.

I'd worked in a Coroner's Office in the past, seeing and hearing some awful things but also knew that I was comfortable with death. When a temporary job came up to work in Bereavement Services attached to a hospital, I applied. As soon as they knew I'd worked at the Coroner's Office, I was interviewed on the same day and I felt a sense of belonging from the start.

After the interview, the Manager of Bereavement Services and I had a chat in the family room. This is a small seating area where the family of the deceased collect paperwork or wait before viewing the body. There was a double door to the office, covered with blinds that led to the viewing room. Through that was another door which took you to the Mortuary itself.

"Do you want me to show you around?" asked Wendy, the manager. An undertaker had just dropped a body off and I could see it through the doors as the blinds were open. I realised at that point that there's a human instinct to say, "I'm so sorry." There was no-one to say "sorry" to. Neither Wendy nor the undertaker had any link to this person but, from that moment, I was aware of the automatic reactions we have to death in our society.

I'd seen countless dead bodies at the Coroner's Office so that side of things wasn't shocking or upsetting to me. I had watched postmortems before and seen police body camera and CCTV footage of suicides. I believed that the body is just a casing, not the essence of someone, it's just the packaging. In fact, it had always fascinated me that you can be here one minute, so entrenched in life, and gone the next.

Within six weeks I was there, working in the Mortuary. That was it, that was my new job – and I had no idea that my life was about to change in ways I could never imagine.

Working at a Coroner's Office, if someone has died in hospital, you have to ascertain their medical background and complete some admin. But in the Mortuary, there was so much more. It wasn't just the paperwork I'd have to collate; I would also be liaising with medical staff, funeral directors, the Registrar's office, and any other agencies that were involved.

Bereavement Services isn't counselling, which is often what people think is suggested by the name. It's more of a signpost for the next stage of the process if someone dies in hospital. I was thrown in at the deep end and there was a lot to take in.

"If a patient passes on the ward, someone, usually a nurse will tell the family to come to us," Wendy told me. "It's the ward staff who do the 'last offices' checklist – this just means the procedures performed to the body of the deceased. They'll confirm that all responses have been tested, such as breathing and reflex. They'll remove any jewellery and, when they come to us, they'll be in whatever clothing they were in when they died."

Next, I had to get to grips with the layout of a medical certificate.

Part One:

1A – the disease or condition immediately causing death.

1B – other diseases or conditions that caused 1A.

1C – any other diseases or conditions that led to 1B.

Part Two:

Other significant, existing conditions contributing to the death.

Wendy went on to explain, "The usual process is that one of the nurses tells the family to contact the Bereavement Office. Someone will explain the process to them and arrange for the collection of the medical certificate. This isn't something they can do immediately, as it takes some time to complete. The body gets sent to the Mortuary via the porters and their notes go with them. The family gets assigned a Bereavement Officer. That's you now, Kate, you're one of the team and you'll be one of their first ports of call.

"In the meantime, you need to go through all the patient's records. Make sure all their details are completed correctly – their full name, the date and time of death, that sort of thing. Then you need to go through the notes. Document the names of any doctors who treated them during their last admission, so that someone involved in their care while they were alive can offer a cause of death.

"Start at the end and work backwards, so that you're contacting the doctors who had the most recent input. Go through everything – check if they've had any falls, operations or procedures that might have contributed to their death, as these cases need to go to the coroner. The next of kin have five days to come to the office, collect the paperwork, register the death, and there's a lot to do in that time."

My head was spinning already. This was all stuff that happened in the background when someone died, things that people didn't really have any awareness of but that were vital to the process.

Wendy had more to tell me. "Sometimes, you can't get someone to do the certificate because it's just mobbed up on the wards. There are lots of locums, especially in A&E, and they can be even harder to track down. The doctors

4

might not even remember the patient as they're so busy, which means we need to get as much in order as possible."

"And, when people come here – what happens then?" I asked.

"They'll obviously be upset – although you can never predict reactions – and some of them are confused about what we even are. We're a 'holding' Mortuary not a 'working' Mortuary, but a few have got their ideas from *Silent Witness*. They think there's all sorts of forensic stuff going on here, that we're chopping people up and solving murders. You'll hear lots of weird things and people have strange assumptions at times. Once they know it's entirely up to them whether they want to see the body, that does help."

I tried not to have any expectations but I've always had an interest in death – hardly anyone wants to discuss it and it's often shrouded in mystery. Now I was in the centre of this veiled world and all I could hope to do was put people at ease, to help them through such a trying time and to offer support.

Wendy interrupted my thoughts. "Another thing – people often don't even want to hear the words 'die' or 'death' or 'dead'. They'll say, 'passed away' or 'gone over' and that's fine, they can use whatever words help them, but you need to make sure they know what's happened."

"They'll know, surely? They're in a Mortuary!"

"Grief does funny things. I've lost count of the number of times I've had to emphasise that the person is dead. You can't always use other words. You'll have to say, "When

X is dead, this will happen," or "Now that X is dead." It sounds harsh, but there are people who just won't accept it unless you're really factual. It doesn't mean that you're cold, it just means that they need to know this is it – there's no coming back."

It did sound a bit cold but it wasn't long before I realised the truth of it. People use so many euphemisms to soften the subject, because we hide death in our society, we don't have conversations about it until we're forced to, which for me, is a very unhealthy approach. However, on that first day, before I'd met anyone, I was just taking it all in.

"Remember – they don't have to see the body but neither do you. You can have as much or as little involvement with the Mortuary as you like. It's up to you."

I nodded but I'd made my mind up. This was something I knew I could do and I already felt at home.

It was vital that I familiarised myself with the viewing room as well as all of the other workings of the Mortuary. I wanted to be prepared to answer any questions and be comfortable with the whole set up. It would be awful if someone who was grieving felt that I was some sort of amateur.

"Just pop a pillow under their head and a blanket over them," said Wendy. "The other covers get draped over the sides so that the family, or whoever is viewing, doesn't get too upset by thinking it's all very clinical."

On that first day, I concentrated on learning how to arrange everything perfectly. I was told that the body had to be covered up to mid-chest so that the family could see their neck and face. Obviously, there were going to be cases where this wasn't practical: for instance, I knew that a young girl had been in the day before who had been hit on the side of the motorway. Her skull had completely caved in and I was warned that, with similar cases, I'd have to be a bit more strategic with the sheets.

"Will people really want to do a viewing if someone has died like that?" I asked.

"They have to be allowed to see them if they wish – even if we advise them that it could be traumatic," said Wendy.

It was always up to the family. The only thing we could do, along with the police and the Coroner's Office, was to be completely honest about what they would see and advise against it, as much as we might want to scream, "No – don't do it, you'll be haunted forever!"

I could expect the majority of viewings to last about 30 minutes to an hour, but there might be some people who hardly stayed and others who wanted much longer. The viewing room itself had nothing but chairs and a small vase of flowers – until the covered trolley was brought in. It was an unadorned room, a blank slate for the story that would be told, the regrets, the love and the grief which would play out within it.

I would meet the family outside of the viewing room, take their names and their relationship to the deceased, and then show them in. If the body was under the "care" of the Coroner, then the visit would have to be supervised, otherwise the visitor or visitors could be left alone.

I'd been given as much information as I could absorb for the time being and it was time to do my first viewing. Thrown in at the deep end, the family who walked in had lost their grandma. It was a straightforward death – the old lady had been ill before she came into hospital and died quite quickly in the final stages of cancer, before anyone had a chance to organise hospice care. There was a clear cause of death and no need for the Coroner to be involved. It was a mixed blessing really as she'd been in a lot of pain.

As soon as they came in and I walked over, the words came out of my mouth without thinking. *I'm so sorry for your loss.* It's what we all say, isn't it? An automatic expression, a cliché really, but from the first time I uttered it, and for every viewing from that moment on, I meant it. I was sorry, I did feel that their loss needed to be acknowledged immediately.

I wasn't affected in a bad way at all by that first viewing. Everyone in the family – the woman's two sons, a daughter-in-law and a grandson in his 20s – wept, but they also seemed to process it very well. They were really just there to say goodbye, there were no dramatics, no recriminations, nothing more or less than a final farewell to a loved one. They thanked me when they left and I was satisfied that they had got what they needed from it. They were appreciative and respectful, and I suppose I expected that to be the case with every viewing that was going to happen. I didn't dwell on anything but I did empathise. I had, of course, lost loved ones myself but I wouldn't be able to compare every loss to someone I cared for or I wouldn't

8

be able to function. I guess that being in the middle of death like that can focus your mind, but you also need a degree of distance or you'd be bawling your eyes out constantly for what had been lost in your own life and the losses that were to come, too.

As that day went on and I saw more dead bodies than I'd come across in my life, I soon realised that I wasn't a squeamish person when it came to death. I'd had to grit my teeth – and cover my nose – when dealing with hoarders, but this was a different type of potentially uncomfortable situation and it could have been something I might not have been able to deal with; luckily, it didn't faze me at all.

As my first week went on, I realised how little I knew about this world of the dead. I'd never really thought about it. When anyone I'd known had died, I think – after the initial grief or shock or relief if they had been suffering – most of us move on to the funeral arrangements. We're either organising those ourselves if it's a loved one, or preparing to go to one for friends or acquaintances. Being here brought me into the world in between.

I realised that every single body tells a story, and perhaps that was what I had been drawn to all along. On my second day, the main thing I realised was that, despite people knowing that their loved one has been in a fridge before the viewing, they can still be utterly shocked at how cold they are.

"I can pull the blinds back and let you look through the window first," I offered. "It'll give you an idea of what to expect when you go in to see your mum, or even if it's the right thing to do."

"No, we're fine," the son told me, gruffly. "Just need to get this over and done with."

His wife was more upset, dabbing at her eyes. "It might be better, John," she suggested. "So you're not shocked."

"I'm not going to be bloody shocked, am I? I know she's dead, I know what I'm going to see."

"Well, Mum will look like she's lying in a bed," I went on. "But I do have to warn you that she'll be extremely cold."

He rolled his eyes. "Can we just go in?"

His wife hung back a little more before following him in. He strode over to the body and lifted his mother's hand up, dropping it instantly. "Bloody hell! She's freezing!" he shouted. "What's going on here? She's like a block of ice."

I'm not sure what he thought we'd been up to. I would find out in the days and weeks and months to follow that many people just couldn't take on board how cold bodies would be when their blood was no longer pumping. No matter how much I tried to warn them, no matter how I couched it, the fact that they were touching someone who had been in a fridge since they had died was shocking.

It happened a lot. People would touch the body and be jolted by how it felt to them. You think you know what "cold" means, but until you touch a corpse that has just come out of a refrigerator, you have no idea. It's not just that they've been at a low temperature, it's also that their body isn't generating any heat at all. Additionally, there is often moisture coming out of their skin, which can look like sweat, making it even more shocking when the natural instinct is to touch their face or hold their hand – but they're like ice.

In those early days, I only had "everyday" cases to deal with. I hadn't been warned that there might be other types. Maybe that was for the best! I don't think I ever had a line between what I expected grieving people to do and what I didn't. In my first week, I remember a woman calling up after a viewing and quietly asking, "Do you think you could pop back in and tell her I love her again?"

"Of course I can!" I told her. "I'll do that right now and you call me back in five minutes so I can let you know it's done."

I'd never lie to someone about things that are important to them like that. There's no rulebook about how to grieve, and nor should there be. If someone needs something and I can help them, why wouldn't I? My colleagues were the same – we don't want anyone to leave with questions unanswered, with their imaginations running riot. Our respect doesn't end until the body leaves the Mortuary.

After a little while, still in my first month, I'd hover at the start of the viewing as everyone tends to have questions – and if it looked as if they weren't going to follow the rules, I'd hover for even longer. The main issue which arose was the number of people who wanted to take pictures. That – obviously – isn't allowed at all. Yet there would be some who insisted it was a perfectly normal thing to do, and that I was being ridiculous for saying we couldn't let them.

"Where's the harm?" pushed one man. "She's dead – she doesn't know; and she wouldn't mind anyway."

"I'm really sorry, but it's against our rules," I repeated.

He thought about it for a minute. "FaceTime? That'll be OK, won't it? Just let her grandkids have a look."

He wasn't the first to suggest that and a lot of people do it covertly. With one family of 12, they were adamant there were dozens of other relatives who wanted to see the poor woman. They agreed to stick to the rules but, when I left to answer the phone, I got back to see them all with their phones out, snapping away, some of them posing at the side of her. It bewilders me why anyone would want to do that, but maybe it's a sign of the times.

"Why can't we do it?" they would ask.

"It's not appropriate," I'd reply.

"Why?"

"It's about dignity and respect; he can't consent."

"But the family wants to see what he looks like now, whether he looks different."

He looked dead, that's how he looked!

The very next one after the FaceTiming family was the complete opposite. It was a case that was with the Coroner as an unexplained death. A young woman of only 25 had been found unresponsive in her bed that morning. Anyone who came in and was the same age as one of my kids hit hard, and this one was heart-breaking. Her mum wanted to see her that lunchtime, less than four hours after she had been found, and the police warned us that we'd have our work cut out as the mum had severe mental health problems.

"You're new, aren't you?" the officer said to me. "You'll have to watch her. She's volatile and can't be left on her own. Supervise her the whole time, the *whole* time."

I agreed that I would and prepared myself. The body wasn't in a bad state. We knew that she'd had a history of drug use but the police hadn't seen any evidence of an intentional overdose when they found her.

Her mum was broken from the moment she walked in – staggered in, really. I don't think she could even believe where she was. I walked towards her and she fell into my arms.

"Lucy! Lucy! Lucy" she wailed.

"Come on love, let's have a sit down for a moment." I guided her to a chair and sat beside her.

"Is she here?" she asked me, through gulps of tears. "Is she somewhere in here?"

"She is. She's just in that room there." I nodded my head in the direction of the viewing room. "You can see her if you like, or you can just sit here for a bit. It's entirely up to you."

"I want to be with her! I want to be with my Lucy!"

I helped her up – I honestly thought she was about to collapse – and we walked through together. I'd arranged Lucy on the trolley with the usual covers and drapes, a cushion behind her head. She looked much younger than her years, at peace from what I'd been told was a chaotic life. Lucy's mum started screaming with a ferocity that must have been heard throughout the whole building.

With an energy I didn't think she had, the mum ran over to her daughter, grabbed her shoulders and kissed her. She shouldn't even have been touching the girl as, technically, her body was evidence, but it's natural instinct for a mum. She was climbing on the bed, tearing handfuls of her own hair to put in her daughter's hands, and snatching some from Lucy's head, too.

"I'm here Lucy, I'm here!" she kept saying, over and over. I think she wanted to climb on top of her to hold her, but, as I've said, the body is on a trolley even if it looks like a bed – and it moves. I had to stop her before she did that but she pushed me off. The poor woman was delirious, shouting and screaming, weeping and wailing. It was beyond anything I'd dealt with yet.

All of a sudden, she ran towards the door.

"I can't do this, I have to get out," she told me.

"Where are you going to go?"

"Does it matter? Lucy's gone and I don't want to be here either."

She wasn't in any fit state to go anywhere. I got her to sit back down again and called Wendy, who was in a different part of the building.

"I can't allow her to walk off by herself," I said. "She could do anything."

Wendy came in and, after a quick chat, agreed. She phoned the Psychiatric Ward and asked if someone could come down and chat.

"No," she was told. "It's not our job to do that."

"But she's distraught – she's breaking her heart."

"It's not our domain. She's got capacity."

Wendy pushed and pushed, and they eventually came down to the Mortuary. After about 30 seconds, the Psychiatrist said, "she's fine," and left. I talked to that poor woman for ages as I was incredibly concerned that she'd have to go home by herself. She kept crying as she told me about Lucy, how she'd been her world and that life revolved around her. She registered absolutely nothing I said. She just wanted to talk about Lucy. It was disjointed and grief stricken, and her behaviour made me sure she'd jump in front of the next bus.

All of a sudden, she stood up. "I have to go now."

"Can you call someone? Is there a friend who could sit with you for a while? I really don't think you should be on your own," I said.

"I've been alone all my life," she sighed. "All I had was Lucy." Finally, she agreed to call a neighbour. Just as she was walking out of the door, she turned to me.

"I want her to have something. I want Lucy to have something nice."

"Do you have something you'd like me to put in with her?" I asked.

She shook her head. "Not really. She's my little girl – I just want her to have something to keep her company."

I looked at that poor woman and thought of my own daughter. I fought back the tears that were threatening to come – this wasn't my grief and it would be wrong to push that on her. "I could get her a teddy, would you like that?"

She nodded and I kept my word. Lucy's mum came back for one more visit – with a police officer this time, so I don't know what had gone on since she'd left the day before, and it was none of my business. She seemed more resigned, but still lost. And why wouldn't she be?

Another case that really hit home for me was the death of another young woman. She was only 18 and had been found dead on the motorway. It was a Saturday night when she came in and, when I opened the body bag six hours after she'd been found, the stench of alcohol hit me like a wall. I was sure that was why she'd died, there was so much of it still in her. The police claimed that she'd been involved in some drug trafficking and believed her death was gang-related, with it being most likely she'd been kicked out of a car, drunk. When they looked at the CCTV and pieced it together, that hadn't been the case at all. This poor girl – Rachel – had indeed been drunk and was hitch-hiking to get home. She lost her balance and was hit by a car, which drove off.

It shouldn't matter who it is, but when they're the age of your kids, the family reaction hits you. Rachel's mum said she was the quiet one, the free spirit who was always travelling. I was starting to get a real sense of who these people were, the ones who ended up with us. It was really poignant when all I had known of them up until that point was their body, but then the family would often tell stories and show photographs, breathing life into them again.

I realised very quickly that this was a job that suited me. I had stumbled upon it but it was the first time during my working life that I actively enjoyed coming into work. It was a home from home. Normal in my new workplace was macabre and unusual; you can't be unsympathetic or desensitised, but you are also dealing with a world that very few people know anything about.

In my second week, I was told about pacemakers. Anything electrical has to be removed from the body as it will explode during cremation, which includes pacemakers; they can be switched off during burials though. I watched as Wendy talked me through it.

"You can often see where the skin is thinner on the chest where it's been inserted," she told me. "If there's more flesh there, you should be able to feel the shape – it'll be about the size of an egg, but flatter. Make a small incision like this…" She ran a scalpel along the top edge, about 1cm or so. "Pop your gloved up finger in and scoop it out. It'll still be attached to the wiring, so cut those off, poke them back in, and sew it all up again. They all go in a box over there as they get recycled. You can do the next one."

I found that fascinating. The pacemaker had been keeping the person alive but it didn't know they were now dead, so it would constantly be trying to reset the heart. I can barely sew a button on but, from the start, I concentrated hard to make a neat wound. There was a moment in my first one where I thought, *I hope I'm not hurting you*, and that notion never went away.

Some bodies seemed almost perfect, even in death, with not a blemish or mark on them – in stark contrast to one man who came in at the end of the month who was absolutely covered in tattoos. There was barely an inch of Keith that didn't have an inking. An array of names and dates of birth (I guessed), trees, lyrics, and things I couldn't quite make out covered his legs, arms, chest and back. "You're giving me quite a show here, Keith," I chatted to him, as I prepared him for his viewing. They were fascinating, they really were, and had obviously been done over many years as you could see the different stages of the ink, in some places darker than others, in some places quite faint green.

Keith's wife and three children came in to view him. He was only in his 50s, and they were in bits. When his wife, Carol, went over to hold his hand, she laughed. "Look at him!" she said. "Every time he went out, I thought he'd come back with another one. What will I look at now Keith? What will I look at now? Do you know," she said to me, "he's got everyone he every loved tattooed on his body in one way or another. His mam and dad, our kids, me, a little one we lost… That man was a walking treasure chest of memories. Here, Leon," she called to her son who was standing behind her. "Show the lady what you got!"

Leon didn't need any further prompting. He rolled up his sleeve and I could see, behind a thin layer of clingfilm, his dad's image tattooed on his upper arm. "Went out straight away and got that," he said proudly. "My first one – only wish Dad could have seen it."

"He knows, love," said Carol. "He knows."

It was honestly one of the most genuine and loving interactions I'd had so far. Keith had clearly been as loved as he'd loved others – and I'd put money on Leon carrying on the tradition.

I'd already learned that people were at the lowest point of their life when they walked into that viewing room, but I'd still seen such goodness in them – and Keith's family fitted that description. People would call days later to say, "Thank you". They would bring in chocolates and send flowers, and they would show such gratitude that they were allowed to say one last goodbye. I focused on that. It was a privilege to be able to facilitate something so poignant that it could make the difference between someone being able to come to terms with their loss or else never being able to move on.

The different ways in which people approached it was an endless source of fascination. Some didn't have much to say, they just wanted one last hug or kiss; some didn't even want to touch, they just wanted to look and say goodbye; others wanted to say sorry for past events or some needed to sit and reminisce about all the special times they'd shared; some never made it through the door at all. But for everyone, it was about getting to grips with exactly what the person had meant to them, whether that was for better or worse. There seemed to be a closure and clarity in getting feelings off their chest and saying what was in their heart for one last time. I knew I'd made the right decision to come here, it was somewhere I already felt at home – and I was sure I would learn lessons about life every day I spent amongst the dead.

Chapter 2
June 2019

I knew that we would get babies in the Mortuary and, honestly, I had no idea how I would cope with that. I felt that I was doing quite well, I always tried to be compassionate yet professional... but babies? That was going to hit hard. When Wendy talked me through this aspect of our work, I initially thought it would be about little ones who were stillborn or had suffered cot death. I didn't realise that we would also get premature births and terminations.

"There are different sizes of things for the baby viewings," Wendy told me. "Someone donated a beautiful Silver Cross pram which is for full-term or stillborn little ones, then a range that goes down to a normal wooden cot, some bassinettes, and there's a wicker basket with a hood that's about the size of a loaf of bread. We use those the most." *The most.* There was so much loss hidden in those words. All of those shattered hopes and dreams wrapped up in a baby who didn't make it and was now with us.

"Then we have small ice cream tubs that have been lined with fabric and made into tiny cots with dolls pillows. There's also a miniature clasped jewellery box which is about the size of a pack of cigarettes, not much bigger than a bar of soap really, with a little tiny pillow and cover that were made to fit."

I found out that there were groups of ladies who made the bedding and also the drawers full of clothes to dress them in. I had no idea what their own stories were, but I could imagine that many of them had been through this too. There were gowns, hats, shawls, even tiny sleeping bags with ribbons. The hats were in every colour of the rainbow, and were vitally important because, if the baby had died on the ward and a little hat had been popped on, mums would want to take that home with them. They smelled of their baby which meant we would change them into new ones from what we had in our store. There were so many options, even some packaged clothes which had been bought from a company that specialised in clothing for premature babies. Some of those outfits are used the most often and they can be very elaborate – suits with waistcoats, elaborate embroidered dresses. They're deliberately not generic, not just a pile of white gowns; they help to give an identity to each little bundle.

I soon found out there would be occasions when mums would come down from the ward to choose clothes in advance and that I would dress their baby for the viewing. I just wanted them to look nurtured and cosy.

My first experience was with twins, one boy, one girl. They were only 18 weeks gestation and one of them was smaller than the other. Their mum had miscarried for no obvious reason and the little girl had taken a breath when she was born. This is quite common. Often, when a premature baby is born, a gasping noise is heard. It's not always a true respiratory breath but, if it's noted as such, it changes the status of the baby from being stillborn to having been born alive, even if only for a few seconds or minutes.

I wanted to look after these babies. I know it might sound perverse, but it seemed like the natural thing to do, it was a way to show that I cared. I knew their mum was coming for a viewing and I was determined to make it something that would be as... well, not as easy as it could be, as it was a horrific situation, but I would do what I could. I treated them as I would my own babies. They were tiny, of course, but also perfectly formed. Often twins don't develop so well in the womb as a single pregnancy, but this little pair was perfect, they even had their tiny little nail beds. I dressed one in pink, one in blue, being gentle and careful with their little heads, holding them just as I would live babies, wrapping them up in soft blankets. When I looked at them, when they were dressed, my immediate instinct was to rock them in my arms; and I did. I felt terribly sad that they wouldn't have their lives, but I couldn't become upset in front of their mum, she was dealing with enough. Crying in that sort of situation might be a natural response, but it would also be a selfish one when you're faced with someone else's pain.

I put them in a bassinet, one at either end, with a tiny little teddy for each baby. All of these things are an attempt to make a very unnatural situation look normal. When their mum came to see them, she was obviously upset and didn't talk. I left her with them – she was on her own with no-one to support her – and when she came out after an hour or so, she just gently whispered, "Thank you" and left.

People's emotions do always get to you but all you can do is give them that space to grieve and let them see that their loved ones were given respect and care until the very end. With babies, I discovered quite quickly that it's almost always just the mums – maybe the men don't want to do it or have a different way of processing their feelings. Or maybe the women want to be alone, I don't know. I do think there is an element of, *You alone have carried them and now you alone have to let them go.* It's the most unnatural experience in the world.

That second month, amongst the pain and heartache of that poor woman losing her two babies, I also had my first introduction into how death can bring out the worst in people. Death can bring people together, but it can also highlight toxic streams running through entire families. When my own sister died, it made me realise just how short life is and what matters and what's important. I guess some people never get that clarity.

"You got my dad in there?" were the words that came straight at me when I answered the phone one morning.

I was taken aback. "Good morning – if you can give me some details, I'll try and help you."

"Gordon Matthews," snapped the young man on the other end of the line. "Just heard he died a couple of days ago. You got him?" I asked for some more information such as his full name, his date of birth and when he had died. I needed to know the family dynamics – was he married, divorced, who was the eldest child? – so that I could establish who was the legal next of kin. Regardless of the fact there are very limited details that can be given out over the phone, it could be anyone at the other end and you can't risk giving away confidential information.

He gave me some details and then added, "I just want to let you know, if you let that bitch he was shacked up with in there to see him, you'll regret it. They're not married, she isn't next of kin – I am. I mean it. If you let her in, you won't know what's hit you."

I confirmed that we had his dad with us, but it wasn't enough to stop him ranting some more.

"They've only been together five years – she's got no right to anything. We're dealing with this, not her. She's not to see him, she's not to know the funeral date. She's to know nothing."

I didn't feel that there was much point asking him if he was sure, as he didn't sound like he was much in the mood for compromise, so all I could do was ask when he would like to come for a viewing.

"A viewing? Why would I want to come and see that piece of shit?" he roared. "I don't want to see him, my sisters don't want to see him – just keep that bitch away from him."

It turned out that Gordon's partner had been with him when he died, and she'd actually called his son to let him know, despite knowing that they all hated her. They blamed her for their parents' marriage breaking up and were doing all they could to twist the knife now. There was nothing we could do. She wasn't allowed a viewing. We checked with the hospital's legal department, but the rules were clear. It was hopeless for that poor woman, on top of her grief, she was completely cut out of everything to do with the passing of the man she loved.

It was a realisation of how bitter people can be. I tried to reason with the son but he was set – and smug now that he had some power and control. I was finding out that rather than bringing people together, some use death to score a few petty points.

Family and friends were quite surprised by what I was doing. They'd thought it would purely be an admin role, not death and corpses, but they could also see that I was really enjoying what I was doing for the first time in a long while. Certain questions and issues came up frequently; there were things people clearly wanted to say or ask but were unsure about how they could approach it, or even if it was appropriate.

There was often a concern about postmortems. They weren't something performed by us but I had watched several take place whilst at the Coroner's Office. That experience meant I knew all about the process and could try to reassure families that it was all done very respectfully. Of course, it's something that plays on your mind, the thought of your loved one being cut into, opened up for answers, their body laid out to try and figure out the story of their death. Apart from postmortems, there were some other questions which came up time and time again.

Will they be cold?
Will they be lonely?
Is it dark at night?

None of these questions are silly, they are things which come into our minds when we're in the middle of grief. When people ask these questions, they're still thinking of their loved one as the person they knew and adored, with the same hopes and fears – notions like loneliness and cold and fear of the dark are actually perfectly understandable.

A lot of misunderstandings came from TV programmes, especially American ones.

Do you glue their eyes shut?
Do you sew their mouths closed?
Do you do their hair and make-up?
Do they sit up?

The answer was *No* to all of that. Funeral directors did most of it and there wasn't a secret room with every single body laid out on marble slabs. I distinctly remember one woman who had a list of questions she'd brought in, not just hers, but everything her family wanted to ask – from the dark tone of the questions, some were also from curious acquaintances, it would seem.

Behind it all, she was terrified. The thought of her beloved husband in there, a sudden death from a heart attack in a fit and healthy man in his early forties, that no-one could have predicted, had left her struggling to hold onto some sense of reality.

"Will he be in there on his own?" she asked me before the viewing.

"Yes, when you go in – which is just in your own time – it'll just be your husband there," I told her.

"No – I mean when I'm not there, when I leave him. Where is he? Is he in a room by himself?"

"He's cared for in the Mortuary just behind us," I replied, trying to not say any words which were harsh.

"He's in a freezer, isn't he? You've frozen him."

"No, not a freezer – just a temperature-controlled environment." I desperately tried to be diplomatic, not entirely comfortable stating cold, hard facts (pardon the pun).

"On his own?"

"Not on his own, there are lots of other patients there, too, and the team is here all day," I explained.

"He'll be cold when you touch him – if you want to touch him," I said, gently. "We do have to keep everyone at a certain temperature."

"Is he embalmed?"

"No – no, we don't do that."

"Do you need to? Do you think you should? Does he need it? Will you do it when I leave?"

"No. We don't do anything like that. They are the decisions you'll make with your funeral director. We'll just look after him until you make all the arrangements that are needed."

She stopped for a moment, nodding.

"Would you like to go in now?"

"Maybe… Do you ever see them move? Once they're here. Have you ever seen someone move and… you've got it wrong, they're not dead? Have you ever seen that? You do hear about it happening." I shook my head. This poor woman was desperate. "You will make sure he's dead? I couldn't bear the thought of him getting buried alive – but I want him back, I really do want him back." The tears started to flow even harder and I put my arm around her.

"I'm so sorry, but he really has gone. I'll make sure he's treated with the utmost respect and you can stay with him as long as you want to – but he has died. There's no other way to say it."

People want tiny details, but they have seen so many horror stories on TV that lodge in their minds and shape their ideas. They think you'll mess with the body, make fun of them, take photographs for WhatsApp groups, all sorts of macabre imaginings – and they often verbalise these thoughts just to get them out there.

Asking us if the person is really dead is quite common. I'd heard it a few times since I'd started work there and, although it might seem ridiculous, it's just the last gasp of hope. Maybe, maybe, maybe… Especially if the person has died without a preceding illness or they aren't very elderly. If their death is beyond comprehension, why would them coming back to life not be possible?

They're often embarrassed to ask, or they don't want to ask in front of anyone else − but the truth is, whatever they *do* ask has been raised a hundred times before. One man specifically came out of a family viewing to seek me out.

"Can I ask you something?" he began. "Where do you take the body after this?"

"Well, the funeral director will come and collect your loved one once everything is arranged and the paperwork is in place."

"No, I mean before that. Where do they go?"

I had no idea what he meant and, whilst I was trying to figure it out, he narrowed his eyes at me suspiciously as if I was keeping something from him. "You're claiming they go nowhere else? No-one else has access to them. Is that right?"

I nodded.

"I see, I see," he said, then walked back into the viewing room.

Some people want to cleanse themselves, to get things off their chest, whether those things are good or bad. Other people want reassurance that the funeral director they've chosen is a nice person. There are also families who have worries on top of their grief and simply don't know how they'll pay for it. This was something I would see more and more of as time went on. One man whose dad had died had three daughters, all of whom were disabled in one way or another.

"I want him buried," he told me at the viewing. "He can't be cremated, he'd hate that." Of course, this is entirely up to the family, but burials tend to cost significantly more than cremations and this man simply didn't have the money given all his other commitments. Fridge space is precious but, if a family can't pay for things to move on, we can't exactly kick them out. This poor man needed at least £5,000 for the send-off he had in mind for his dad but, in reality, he only had £200. The deposit alone was £1000. We didn't hear from him for ages. Phone messages went unanswered and, I suspected, like so many others in the same position, he was just hiding his head in the sand. He must have been torn between giving a service that he knew was against his dad's wishes or doing the only practical thing he could afford. Finally, weeks after his dad had died, the son called me, elated.

"I've got the money!" he told me.

"Oh, that is good news," I replied. "It'll be a comfort to be able to lay your dad to rest and move forwards."

"Yes," he said, and I could hear him sigh with relief. "That's the deposit sorted – just the other four grand to find."

Only the deposit! His dad was with us for months and I finally had to tell him, gently, that the body was deteriorating. I don't know how he finally got the money, it wasn't my business, but he did. I suspect an awful lot of people go into an awful lot of debt just to give the send-off they feel is expected and does their loved one justice.

All of these experiences were giving me some clarity. I was starting to see that some of the things we get hung up on just don't matter. When I'd lost my sister, I had vowed to make changes in my life. I think many of us do that when someone close dies, but maintaining it when life throws other things at you, is hard. I was seeing patterns within the grief. How love presented itself in death, how families reacted to losing someone, how the way we are in life writes the final chapter.

One thing which came up frequently was people saying that they had only "popped out for a minute" or "just gone to the loo" after days of watching their mum or dad or partner towards the end, and yet that was when they had passed. I started to wonder if there is actually some way in which people can die when they want to, whether there is a small part of control at the very end. Families can watch for days, leave the room or the bedside for seconds, and it happens. Maybe it's the last act of love – sparing someone you love the agony of seeing you take a final breath.

There were moments of brevity – lots of them. We were a close-knit team who shared a unique world and got on well as people. A dark sense of humour was essential. We had to have a laugh amongst ourselves, though never at the expense of the people resting with us.

One day I heard Wendy on the phone, breezily saying, "All right my love, see you later. Bye. See you soon, see you!"

"Who's that then? Got a friend visiting you this afternoon?"

"Ah – you haven't met Gareth yet, have you?" she laughed. "Oh, you're in for a treat! He's coming in today and he's going to love you!"

"Who's Gareth?"

"Gareth is our little friend – well, he's huge really – who wants to join our gang. He's adorable, but he's bloody hard work."

Gareth had accosted Wendy in the car park one day, asking her when the bodies were coming. He desperately wanted a job in the Mortuary but was probably the worst person in the world to work there, given that he was unusually keen on it. He came in most weeks and asked the same questions over and over again. Today, he could give everyone else a break and ask me! I'd been off on each of his other visits, and he'd been a bit put out when he'd heard someone else had been taken on, when he was eagerly waiting for his chance.

When he arrived, he launched straight into questions.

"Do you like it, Katie, do you like it here?" he wanted to know.

"I do, Gareth. Everyone has been really nice to me, and it's very interesting."

"It'll be Hallowe'en soon, Katie, won't it?"

"Well, not really. It's a fair bit away." It was June! "Do you like Hallowe'en?"

"I do. I like all the ghosts and skeletons and things. It'll be Hallowe'en soon," he repeated. "What are you doing for Hallowe'en?"

"Nothing really. What are you doing?"

"Nothing probably," he said, sadly. "Are you sure you don't do anything?"

"I keep some sweets at the door in case any kids come trick or treating."

Gareth didn't look happy with that. "Have you ever thought about hiding in the fridges here?" he wanted to know. "For Hallowe'en?"

"Well, I haven't worked here at that time of year before but, no, I'd never hide in the fridges." Then as an afterthought, I quickly told him, "You shouldn't hide in fridges either! Ever!"

"Can I open one and see if I would fit?" he asked.

Wendy was in silent stitches of laughter behind Gareth and I could only imagine how many times she'd gone through all of this before. "Gareth. You can't go in a fridge," she said. "We've had this discussion. You're never, *never*, going in a fridge. Why don't you go along over to the canteen and have a cup of tea?"

She was definitely trying to distract him, as we had tea, coffee and biscuits galore in the office.

"No, I don't want to do that. I want to stay here and talk to Katie," he told her.

"It's almost Christmas," he told me. He'd been talking a while, but it was still June as far as I could tell! "What do you do at Christmas, Katie? What do you do here in the Mortuary?"

"I only started here last month, Gareth. I haven't had a Christmas yet."

"Will you get them all out of the fridges and sing carols to them?"

"I doubt it, I really doubt it."

Gareth wasn't to be deterred. "What's back there?" he asked.

"It's the viewing room," interrupted Wendy. "You know it's the viewing room, you've been in."

"Can I go in now?"

Wendy shrugged at me. "It's empty," she said. "Take him in if you like." It was like she'd given him a winning lottery ticket. He was in there quicker than a rat up a drainpipe.

"What's that?" he asked.

"A frame for a trolley – you must have seen one if you've been in before?"

"Why is it pushed to one side?"

"We're not using it."

"Does the body go there?"

"Not on a frame, no." He started pushing it about.

"Do you put blankets on it? What do I do with the blankets?"

"You do nothing with them. It's not your job," I told him.

"It could be though, I could work here. I wonder why you got the job instead of me?" he mused. I couldn't possibly imagine! "Can I look through in the Mortuary?"

"No, that's only for staff. You must know that?"

"That's why I want a job here. Then I can do all of that. Do you like working here, Katie?" he asked again. "Have you ever put someone in the fridge while they're still alive?"

"No, that doesn't happen."

Gareth scoffed. "It does, I've seen it on telly."

I finally managed to usher him out, only for Wendy to tell me he came for a visit most weeks. I'd just happened to miss him up until that point. There was no harm in letting him into an empty room with only a frame in there, as it satisfied his curiosity and meant that he wouldn't turn up unannounced when we had viewings. He was innocent enough, I think, but everything we did was with respect and Gareth's presence certainly wasn't in line with that. He couldn't become a permanent fixture and he would never, ever be allowed to see a body or get access to the Mortuary for a game of hide and seek.

What he wanted to know was the nuts and bolts of what went on behind the scenes – and, in that, he wasn't much different from most people. Gareth was a moment of light relief in some ways, and we needed it because there was so much that was awful. I'd heard of decomps – decompositions – when I worked in the Coroner's Office. One of the postmortems that I'd watched there was performed on someone who had lain undiscovered in their flat for around six months before the flies and smell alerted a neighbour. As the horror behind the word suggests, these bodies hadn't been found quickly and had started to decompose. Many of them were unrecognisable or unidentifiable. They would be referred to as BTB ("believed to be"), with their name, sex and age if there was any idea, but some came in with even some of those details missing. Any resemblance to the person they were in life was long gone.

I'd seen photos at the Coroner's Office of people found in houses where they'd been lying for weeks or months, but actually having them in the Mortuary was something else. The smell was on another level. Wendy had told me that we had long termers, people who were still being identified or those who had never been claimed.

A process called Estates Research has to be done if someone has no next of kin to act for them. Researchers are sent the details of the deceased and they check archives and registration systems for living blood relatives. If the hospital released a body without these measures, it would have many implications. Usually, they give it about six months – although there's no time set in stone. The researchers exhaust all avenues and if there is still no-one identified to carry out the funeral arrangements, then the hospital will request authorisation and funding to carry out a "hospital cremation". This is simply a direct cremation to give the deceased dignity and also allow much needed fridge space to be freed up. There's no dignity in decomposition and turning into a green ball of fluff.

There is a list of names, BTBs, of all our occupants on a white board in the Mortuary. I started working there in May and knew that someone had been there since January.

Moss Man.

He wasn't keeping well and had been moved from fridge to freezer. He had a layer of fur, like moss, and if you opened the fridge to deal with someone else, a scattering of green dust came out. People deteriorate at different rates and in different ways, but Moss Man went green and fluffy. His eyeballs had fallen back into his head, he had cavities where they'd dropped back into his skull, and his mouth was wide open. Bodies that are frozen look different to those in the refrigerator – they contract, their features become more sunken.

Moss Man was a long termer, with us way before I got there, but, that month, I saw my first one being brought in from the community. It was a woman who had died in the bath and the hot tap had been left running. She was, effectively, poached. She was on her side a bit and still in her clothes. The cause of death was unascertained but, as she was still dressed, it was assumed to be a suicide.

"Decomp coming in!" announced Wendy. "Air freshener out, she's been in the bath for three weeks."

She was brought to us in a black body bag. I was in the office when the body arrived and the smell hit immediately; the most pungent, rotten, fishy smell – like drains. One side of her body was flat as she'd lain there for so long. Usually everything would pool and become black. However, in this case, the water had almost rinsed away her bottom half but not the top.

Not long after her, came another woman who had been found outside, eaten away by foxes and flies. She was so decomposed that she could barely be contained in the bag and she was slushing about. There were maggots coming out of every orifice. The smell genuinely made my eyes water and I had to quickly master breathing through my mouth with a mask on, which is pretty tricky. She'd only been outside for four days, but because of the hot weather and exposure to the elements, she had decomposed rapidly.

One morning, Harry exclaimed, "We've got a big one coming in!" Whoever it was, we'd have to work fast as there was a viewing that afternoon and everything would have to be ready. "We'll need to rearrange the shelves."

There were a few separate fridges for the bigger bodies, called bariatric fridges. When this woman came in, I could see that she was huge. She was well over six feet tall, but she must have weighed about 25 stone as well. She was extremely wide, her belly was distended and stood proud on her body, not unlike a hill.

"Make sure the family don't touch her tummy," said Harry. "She died of something gastric related and, if they lean on it, whatever's there will come out of her mouth." When the fridge door was open, all you could see was stomach. People often have an instinct to rub someone's tummy or stroke the covers that are on top of the bodies, so I needed to make sure they didn't do that… or there would be an explosion.

It all went well, without any incident, and the woman was clearly very much loved. When it's genuine, you feel it, the love is almost tangible and it's nice to think a life has been filled with affection. People always apologise if they're upset, even though it's the most natural thing in the world. At other times, it was almost a bit contrived, and I'd get the sense that the family members were doing or saying what they thought was expected, as if there is a right way and a wrong way to grieve. The more fractured and fraught relationships appeared to have been in life, the more dramatic the display of grief seems to be at the end – and I'd already seen people throwing themselves on the floor, giving Oscar-worthy performances. All life was condensed there, all human emotions and all human reactions – it was a window to the world.

Chapter 3
July 2019

I felt at home from the start but, as time went on, I realised I actively enjoyed it. I was seeing that attitudes to death vary massively, not just from person to person but from culture to culture. Seeing how different cultures deal with the process of death was enlightening and fascinating.

You tend to see Muslim families only briefly, as they often have a large support network, and their religious requirements are that a burial has to take place quickly in accordance with their beliefs. Most Muslim families would like the body taken to the mosque as soon as possible after death, so that burial can be completed within 24 hours. Unfortunately, hospital processes don't always work like that. Many doctors are sympathetic, others not so much. There are some who fully understand that it's culturally significant and, in those cases, we tend to get a call from the ward to advise us ahead of time, so that we know the clock is ticking. These are commonly called "expedited" cases. We do understand and empathise, and we always move as quickly as possible. But we can't deal with just one case and we can't make miracles happen. Some families can be very forceful and will arrive en masse, believing that you've never faced these demands or situations before – and that you aren't sympathetic to their cause or respectful of their wishes.

In August, I got my first experience of just how much some people want to bend the rules. There was an elderly Muslim man who was in the final stages of his life and expected to die over the weekend. This sounds hard hearted, but the weekend is the most inconvenient time to die if you want a swift release, as there can often be staffing issues. On the Friday, the family asked if a doctor would pre-sign a death certificate, as they wanted all the paperwork ready should he die over the weekend, out of hours. When the legal impropriety of what they were requesting was explained to them, they weren't very happy. They could see no good reason why a certificate could not be completed in advance. Naturally, no-one would do this – and he very considerately lasted until the Tuesday when all his paperwork was dealt with swiftly.

On a busy ward, there can easily be five or six hours between a patient dying and a doctor being available to formally verify the certificate. That can create a huge problem if you want everything done within 24 hours. There was one woman whose son died on his birthday and she didn't want that date on the death certificate. She asked if he could be verified after midnight, so it would go down as the next day. She felt it would taint her memory every year. But it also meant she was torn between legal accuracy and the clock ticking away, leaving an even smaller window for him to be buried.

I also discovered that, in Muslim families, it tended to be the men who dealt with matters. My experience of most other groups was that, more often than not, it was the women who organised everything.

At the start, I put a lot of obnoxious behaviour down to grief but I was starting to see that some people were just bloody rude. I'll never forget the two old ladies who came in like something from the 1970s, real Churchy types with bunches of fake flowers, rosary beads and a crucifix. They acted like butter wouldn't melt and asked if I could give them some time with the body. When I returned, they were FaceTiming his Filipino wife and gave me dog's abuse when I called them out on it, with language like you could never have imagined!

It was August when I had one of my most memorable cases. We had a phone call about a 51-year-old man who had suffered a sudden cardiac arrest. He'd been taken to A&E but was dead on arrival. It was verified by the Coroner and he was brought to us for arrangements to be made. The day after, we got a call from a woman called Maria, who said she was his wife.

"Are you his next of kin?" we asked.

"Yes, I'm down as that." We checked the paperwork, and she was indeed named on it. When Maria got there, we had to warn her that, although her husband, Joe, was perfectly intact, he did still have his breathing tube in.

I stayed with her as that sort of thing can be quite upsetting and watched as she gently stroked his arm.

"I'm so sorry, Joe, I'm so sorry. I'll bring Amy up as best I can."

As she left the viewing room, I asked her what age their little one was. "Just six," she told me. "Just six. I don't know how she'll cope without her daddy." She was so upset. I gave her a cup of tea and we sat together for a while. The next day, I got a call from the Coroner's Office to advise that Joe's wife wanted a viewing.

"That's fine. She's been in already but she can come back."

There was a pause. "OK – well, just to confirm, she will be in to view later today. We've told her about the breathing tube, just as a head's up."

"No problem, she's already seen it."

"Well, she can't have. She hasn't been in."

"She has," I confirmed. "She was in yesterday."

There was another pause. "We're talking about Joe's wife, Rachel. She most definitely has not been in."

It turned out that Maria was not his wife – or his legal next of kin. She was someone he had been having an affair with, while his real wife went through years of fertility treatment to have their two-year-old. Not only would she have to be told that her husband had betrayed her for many years, she would also find out that he had another child. It was actually a police officer who had the harrowing task of telling her all of this. Despite everything, she still wanted to come and see Joe.

I said to Wendy, "God, how awful to learn all of that and get no answers from him." I felt so sorry for Rachel when she came in. She was a tiny, completely broken woman. I took her in to see him and asked if she would like me to stay. Without a word, she walked over to her husband, stared at him for the longest time – then just started punching and punching. I held her and pulled the cord to get help. Wendy and I sat down beside her and just let her get it all out. She was so hurt – and why wouldn't she be? Her life had been a web of lies for years and she was denied the chance to ask the questions which must have been swarming in her head.

"I only came to hit him," she wept. "I bet you think I'm disgusting." I definitely didn't. We never know how those stories end but Rachel would never get closure. The only person who could tell her what had gone on was dead, and she had to face up to everything he had done to her, with no hope of emotional justice.

I see snapshots of life in the middle of death. I see the most dramatic bits of a film but not the ending. Rachel had stood there staring at him, then it was as if she'd been ignited and gone on the attack. That case went to inquest and both his wife and mistress would have to be there. I have no idea what happened but the nightmare wasn't going to be over for Rachel any time soon. I thought about her a lot.

In the midst of it all, there can be moments of such pure love that your heart is lifted. I found that in the story of a Polish couple called Alek and Julia. Julia was only in her early 40s, when she died in the middle of the night after a routine operation in hospital. She came to us and, very soon after her arrival, Alek called.

He was such a polite man. I could hear the absolute agony in his voice when he said, "Please, could I ask you something? We have an eight-year-old son. Should I bring him to see his mother?"

"I'm so sorry," I had to tell him. "We can't be seen to influence anyone, either way. It has to be your decision."

"Does she... does she look scary?"

I offered to go in and see Julia, just to put his mind at rest. Wendy went with me to the fridge. "What do you think?" I asked her.

"She's stunning, isn't she?" she replied. I nodded in agreement; she really was.

"She looks absolutely beautiful," I said when I returned to the phone. I was telling the truth.

"Will my son be frightened?" I wasn't allowed to say – and I didn't know. Some children can cope, others can't. I apologised again for sitting on the fence. "Does she look like she is sleeping?"

"Yes. Yes, she does. Why don't you come alone first? It doesn't have to be just one visit – you can decide whether you think your little boy should come, too, once you've seen your wife."

And that is just what he did. Alek was so sweet with her. He stroked her forehead constantly. "Isn't she beautiful?" He wanted confirmation before he couldn't look at her any longer. Every time he asked, I agreed – no-one could have denied it. "She has never had a line on her face and now she never will." The tears were flowing from his eyes, but he retained such dignity as the love emanated towards Julia. "I just can't... I can't understand how she can be dead. It makes no sense. She's beautiful, isn't she?" he asked again and again.

After a while, he asked if I would like to see a photo of their son. The most adorable boy gazed out at me, with his mother's looks. "Should I bring him?" Alek pressed.

"I can't say, I just can't say."

He thought about it. "I don't think he should remember his mother this way. Maybe if he was older... Who knows? I feel he has been through so much losing her. What if this, seeing her here, was the image which burned through all of the others? Not her face smiling at him, not the way she looked when she read stories to him at bedtime, but this. She is so beautiful still, yes, but she is gone. My Julia has gone."

He never did bring his little boy and I feel he made the right decision, but it would have been completely unprofessional and inappropriate of me to steer him either way.

Some people want to be left alone, they find it intrusive to have anyone else there. When there is a baby, I feel there is a purity in that situation, a love that is completely true. Quite often, we would get calls from a bereavement midwife, irrespective of whether the baby was a 12-week pregnancy, a full-term baby, or a stillbirth. They would call as soon as the loss had been verified and give a brief overview, as well as sending notes with the body.

In August, a little boy came in who was only 14 weeks gestation. He was actually very well developed for that stage and I was coming to realise that the books and the charts aren't always accurate. There is no exact science and there can be huge differences between babies at different stages of development in the womb, just as there are at birth. I could actually see hair on this tiny boy. Doctors had found a genetic abnormality when performing routine tests and his mum had opted for an elective termination. She, Laurie, had spent a lot of time with a bereavement midwife and was distraught. At 14 weeks, many women are just left alone with no support from bereavement services, but because Laurie had been in the system from the start, she had the support and input of the maternity staff.

"She'll want a lot of involvement," the midwife told me. "She'll need a lot of access to him." Laurie had kept her little boy on the ward with her after she'd delivered so he didn't come to us until nine the next morning. The midwife came down with him and said, "She's in bits."

I know that some people will find that hard to understand. She was "only" 14 weeks pregnant and the baby – the foetus really – was tiny. But he was her baby, he was her little boy. Laurie did want a lot of access, she did want a lot of involvement, but she didn't have a baby she could hold and rock. Like everyone who suffers a loss, her grief was unique to her and it can't be minimised by some arbitrary date on a chart or someone deciding at what stage you're allowed to weep for the baby who never was.

You get such insight into the maternal bond with women who have lost their babies. It's still there no matter the age of the baby or the stage of pregnancy. They still want to love, and that is a strength which is incredible, but they also need somewhere for that love to go. Laurie's pain was exacerbated by the fact that this was a decision she'd had to make herself and the feelings of guilt were evident.

There is always a story with any death, but I found the ones with babies particularly poignant – that of Mary and baby Abigail even more so than usual.

"There's a woman who's been on the phone," said Wendy. "Her little one is being brought in this morning first thing and she wants to see her as soon as possible."

That was fine, that was what often happened. Mary was an older mum and had found out during an amniocentesis test that her baby had Down's Syndrome. If she had gone to full term with her daughter, the baby may have had a low quality of life and not survived for very long. Mary had decided to terminate. After a lengthy induced labour, she'd given birth to Abigail in the early hours of the morning. We were ready for Mary by about 11.00am.

She walked in with her head bowed. I thought that she seemed in physical pain, as well as emotional, which was probably the case given that she'd just gone through such a difficult labour.

"I'm so sorry for your loss," I told her. "Would you like to come through with me now to the viewing room, or would you prefer to sit here for a little while?" She just pointed at the door and looked at me, as if to ask whether that was where she needed to go. "Yes, we go in there," I told her.

I'd done all I usually do with Abigail. Although she was so tiny, she had dark hair and eyelashes. It was clear to see that she was a Down's Syndrome baby, and that she was beautiful. I'd popped her in a wicker bassinet and been able to dress her in a little pink floral Babygro, wrapping a white blanket around her. I always had this compulsion to keep them cosy. When Mary saw her, the tears started to flow and all she said was, "Abigail."

I left her for a while but, after a couple of hours, it was clear that Mary wasn't going to come out quickly. "Would you like to stay a little longer?" I asked her.

"Yes please – when do you close?"

"We usually have our last viewing at 3.00pm."

"Can I stay until then?"

Luckily, no-one else was booked in that day, so it was fine. When Mary came out at 3.00pm, she asked, "When do you open tomorrow?"

"9.00am," I told her.

"OK – I'll see you then. Until 3pm." With that, she left.

"What if we get someone else who wants a viewing?" I asked Wendy. "It's quiet just now, but it'll be awful if that happens." How could we prioritise who should be able to spend time with their loved one? It's not for us to determine that a mother seeing her baby is any more important than a family seeing a grandparent. We'd have to play it by ear and deal with it if it happened.

She was there first thing in the morning. I'd come in early to get Abigail out and make sure she still looked nice, and it would be a pattern I stuck to for the next two weeks. Wendy did some of those viewings but for each and every day, Mary was there. She started to confide in me after a while and, as we sat, with her holding Abigail, she told me her story. As I'd thought, she was an older mum, and she'd conceived Abigail through donor insemination. It was her last chance at motherhood, as she was in her early 50s.

"My family thought I was mad to even try," she told me, "but I've always wanted a baby. I've always wanted a little girl." She stroked Abigail's cheek as she spoke. "I don't have many friends and the few I did have drifted away as I went through the process. Actually, I think that might have been for the best – when I found out it had worked, all I wanted was me and my little girl. I couldn't have coped if someone had come at me with negativity and judgment. It was just me and her..." her voice tailed off. "And look at us now."

She was going through all of this completely alone – well, almost. I was determined to be there for as long as she needed me, but these things can't last forever. Love can't stop time and bodies deteriorate no matter what. The problem was, Mary had other ideas.

On the second day of visiting, she turned up with two books. One was full of Winnie the Pooh stories, and the other was *Guess How Much I Love You?*

"Can I read to her?" she asked.

"Of course you can – that's a lovely idea."

Mary read *Guess How Much I Love You?* to her baby girl who was still in the wicker bassinet. When she finished, she laid the book down on the chair next to her and took up the much larger Winnie the Pooh collection.

"I'm going to come and read to her every day," she told me. "I won't let her go until I've finished."

And she kept to her word. We couldn't allow her in for six hours each day, but she would fit round other viewings, coming in when there was no-one there, usually two or three times a day. As soon as a family left, I would clear up and get Abigail ready, knowing that Mary was desperate to get back in. Some nights we stayed until 7pm, we even opened up at the weekend and we were happy to do that for her, happy to give her all the time she needed. I got to know her so well as we sat there having a cup of tea with Abigail and it felt so natural – but the clock was ticking.

"She's been loved more than many children are in their whole lives," I told Mary one afternoon. "It's time to let her go now." I hoped she grasped what I meant. Abigail was changing, that much was clear to see.

"I haven't finished her story," she replied. "I can't leave her until the book has ended."

The baby was deteriorating. She was being moved between competing temperatures many times a day and had started to become grey. Her once beautiful skin was shrivelling, although Mary seemed to be in denial about that. She just saw her baby girl. Her little bassinet was full of things, a tiny teddy from us, a woolly hat, a rabbit that was the same as the one in *Guess How Much I Love You?* and a stripey blanket Mary had knitted. To start with, it had been easy to pretend that this was a "normal" set up. But it was now becoming increasingly difficult.

She finally had to agree that Abigail would have to move to the funeral directors and the service needed to be arranged. On the day before that happened, Mary suddenly asked something that I felt she had been avoiding for the previous two weeks.

"Where does she go when I leave? Where do you take my baby?" I'd been dreading it. "She doesn't stay in this lovely bassinet, does she?"

"Oh, she goes through there," I said, directing her gaze to the other door. I was stalling, really, hoping she wouldn't ask the dreadful questions that were in her mind.

"She goes in a fridge, doesn't she?"

"Well, it's a refrigerated area, Mary. It has to be."

"Can she please stay in this tonight?" She indicated the bassinet and I agreed, although as soon as I did, I felt acutely aware that if Wendy said no, I was going to either go against the rules or accept that I had lied to a grieving mother. Luckily, Wendy is equally committed to helping families and agreed that Abigail could rest in her bassinet in the fridge overnight.

That day, that Friday morning before she was taken away, Mary was waiting with her book at 9.00am. She hadn't finished it – and she never would. She stood staring at Abigail, seeing the baby who was perfect to her, even though it had all gone on for far too long.

"Do you want to dress her?" I asked. "I can help you. You can change her hat and keep that one."

"Can I? Can I touch her?"

It was hard and I had to make sure I held the baby in a very particular way, but I think it was the right choice. I think Mary would treasure those moments where she was able to pretend everything was fine. She took the teddy, the hat, the blanket and the rabbit, and put Abigail in a silky little sleeping bag.

Everything affects you in one way or another, but the sight of that lovely woman and the baby she adored, the two of them together in love on that last visit, will stay with me forever. I could feel the bond between them even though Abigail was no longer there. There was something so special but so haunting about the time they had spent together, with the stories that would never be enjoyed by a baby who could hear them and a woman who had so much love to give but no-one to give it to now.

Abigail was collected by the funeral director that afternoon and Mary didn't see her again until the Monday, the day before she was cremated. I actually wished I could have been with her for that last visit. I felt such affection for her and her baby, and it was hard to think I'd never see them again. We all thought of them on the day of the cremation, sending her a card with our love. It was a true privilege to be involved with that little family of two, and I only hoped that Mary would get some closure from the time she had spent with Abigail.

I was finding that there wasn't much of a grey area in terms of what people wanted from viewings, they either came in and out very quickly, or they stayed to try and get a connection with the deceased in some way. A lot of people wanted all the detail, they stared at them, keeping things going for as long as possible. Of course, the Mortuary is a reminder of death and how we'll all end up, but some people were drawn to it, wanting to know every single aspect of what went on there.

"Rosebud House" – what we're euphemistically known as so that the porters have something gentler to shout across at each other rather than belt out they're off to the Mortuary – had so many secrets and there was a macabre attraction for some people who came to viewings. They asked questions about everything, not just those relating to their loved one. In fact, I had one family, just after Mary and Abigail, where the son made me feel I was playing 20 Questions.

"How many have you got in today? Are the fridges full? What's the worst one? You got any nasty accidents? I read about a suicide yesterday – you got that one?" He was constant – worse than Gareth, which was saying something! He barely looked at his old dad lying there, he was too busy trying to squeeze some morbid gossip out of me.

"I'm afraid I can't talk about any other cases," I told him. "I'm sure you understand that we have to respect confidentiality and treat everyone with dignity. Like your dad…"

He wasn't to be distracted. "I bet you've got some juicy tales, haven't you? Come on! Spill the beans!"

He'd have loved to have heard about the woman who came in just a few days later. The word was that we had a particularly gruesome decomp coming in, not that there's ever a good one. She'd been lying undiscovered not for weeks, but months. The body was unrecognisable. We were anticipating the usual smell – cabbage, drains – and we put out a few extra air fresheners, the heavy-duty ones. The body had only been found in the flat eventually because of the smell, and the heat of the summer had made it even worse.

She had landed face down on one side where she'd fallen, and her arm was stuck out at the side. It had been squashed into the body bag, but when that came in and we opened it, the arm sprung out. She was completely black all over with heavy decomposition, but at the end of this arm were the most immaculate acrylic nails. We jumped back as the arm and hand were both decomposing – as was every part of her – but these beautiful purple nails, sparkling with glitter and tiny jewels, glistening under the harsh light, must have been done just before she died.

One side of her had completely disintegrated but the sight of those nails was what I focused on as we dealt with her body. I don't know why, but I thought back to the inquisitive visitor from the previous week who had said to me when he finally left, "I bet you could write a book..."

I reflected on what it is about death that everyone finds so fascinating yet so taboo. I suppose it's partly that it's the only thing that we are all destined to share and that, as the only animal with the knowledge that our death is inevitable, there is no getting away from it. Not long ago, this lady had sat, having her magnificent nails done. And now she lay here, those same nails the only vaguely recognisable thing about her. Game over.

Is death taboo because people think that if we talk about it, then we're inviting it to happen? Is that it? I've spoken to so many people who never had "the conversation" with their lost loved one and are left desperately trying to work out what someone's wishes would have been. Our true wish is to stay here in some immortal limbo and never leave the ones we love, I guess. But wishing won't make that happen. Preparing for things, discussing things, however unpleasant it might seem, takes a bit of the uncertainty from it and gives you the power to deal with death a bit better.

The longer I was in this job, the more passionately I felt about people facing the issue of dying head on. I contemplated what my own children would face if my number was chosen tomorrow. I don't want "not knowing" for them, I don't want them to have disagreements about what I would have wanted to wear or what hymns I'd want (none!), when they'd also be coming to terms with losing their mum. I hope that time is a long way off but my priority, as with most parents, has always been my children and we do them a disservice by not preparing them for a time that is inevitable. I'm not suggesting we make it a daily topic round the dinner table but I do feel that, as a society, we should work to normalise it and remove the fear. Whatever happens afterwards, if anything, it's true to say that the only thing to fear is fear itself. I've seen that fearing death can stop us living life. I've witnessed that first-hand.

Dealing with death on such a constant basis undoubtedly has an effect on the strongest of people, and I'd be lying if I said that I was any different. For a time, I came to constantly fear the worst in the most innocent of situations. If my children were late arriving, I'd picture them being wheeled in on a trolley. If I had a headache, I pictured the words *Spontaneous intracranial haemorrhage* on my death certificate with my weeping children having to decide what to do with my jigsaw collection (they definitely wouldn't be arguing over them). It became all-consuming and, at that point, I answered my own question. *THAT* was why people don't think about it or discuss it; it makes it too much of a realistic prospect and then it starts to impact your ability to actually live. But that is like saying that it's pointless reading a book because it has an ending – knowing that it ends doesn't make the story any less enjoyable, it should just make us appreciate it all the more while we're reading it.

Chapter 4
August 2019

People get confused between Coroners and Mortuaries. They often ask if they can see a deceased relative at the Coroner's Office, not realising that the body isn't there. I think they are confused by things they see on TV shows, especially the American ones whose system is completely different to ours, not to mention highly glamourised. Those programmes have a lot to answer for.

Every hospital has a Mortuary. The one I worked in was a major one and it wasn't solely a holding Mortuary, it was also attached to a teaching hospital as well. This meant we had a lot of junior doctors who had no idea what went on behind our doors.

Every major hospital used to do their own postmortems. That has changed over time, meaning that some mortuaries are purely holding or storage facilities. The Mortuary technicians still do the handling and remove pacemakers and so on but, in many areas of the UK, the examinations are designated to one particular hospital. This was the case for our Mortuary. All mortuary staff wear scrubs and compulsory steel toe capped crocs for health and safety reasons when moving bodies – they may not be the height of fashion but the residents don't seem to mind.

By now, I was well settled and the main piece of guidance I'd been given when dealing with families was to never provide advice. I would often be asked for recommendations of funeral directors, but I couldn't give my opinion – even though I definitely had favourites and some that I wouldn't even use to bury my budgie.

The other question I was asked a lot was *Should I let X see them?* This usually related to a child, or someone who was elderly, or perhaps in a bad way after losing a spouse of many years. But again, as with the Polish family, I just wasn't allowed to offer an opinion or sway them – and it wouldn't have been right even if I could. The key approach was to empathise but not be tempted to give an opinion. I could, however, understand why they might ask. At such an emotional time, when you are drowning under the weight of the choices you need to make, it's tempting to try and get someone else to make those decisions with, or for, you. You're in the middle of a storm at sea and just want someone to offer you a lifeboat, no matter how tiny.

When it came to reassurance though, I could offer as much of that as they needed. I was asked so many times about the dignity of the dead and I could say, with hand on heart, that we observed that at all times. While they were with me and the rest of the team, they would be treated with the utmost respect. Yes, we could have a laugh at times – we needed that gallows humour when faced with so much sadness and loss – but it was never at the expense of those we cared for.

With the questions I was asked, I could often get a glimpse into the lives that had ended. One woman whose sister had died, told me, "She was so sociable, she loved chatting to people and being with them." There was a pause, which often indicates what they're about to say comes from the heart but they feel I'll see it as daft. I never do. "Is she in a fridge on her own?"

I knew she wasn't wondering if her personal space was being invaded and could see that the question was coming from a place of worrying that her sister would be lonely. I never want to give a level of detail that makes anyone uncomfortable. "We can hold up to 120 dead people here!" I told her. "And the Mortuary is full at the moment, so she isn't on her own. We all wish everyone good morning and good night."

"Oh, that's brilliant! She never liked silence." Those few words said so much and she was genuinely placated.

I could still be shocked by the grisly questions of others. From the start, I had been hit with the effects of expertise gleaned from nothing but television and films, and that was showing no signs of abating. There was one man whose mouth was open and we couldn't have closed it without breaking his jaw. He looked like a waxwork – different people become different colours in death, and this man was alabaster white. A lot of cancer patients have skin that becomes very thin and transparent at the end, and it tends to go waxy if they're of white ethnicity. With Asian and Afro Caribbean skin, there is less of a noticeable difference.

Some want a grisly level of detail and you wonder why. One woman whose Dad's mouth was open was transfixed at the sight of him. She recognised that it wasn't completely healthy but kept saying, "I just can't take my eyes off him." He looked like a waxwork and was deathly white. That can make it surreal. "Why isn't his mouth shut?"

"Everyone's face sits differently," I explained.

"Why isn't it shut?" she kept asking, as I gave her the same answer again.

"He's sweating – why?"

"It's not really sweat, it's just little beads of water." I hoped that would be enough for her, I didn't want to explain that it was because he'd been in the fridge and the change in temperature had caused it.

She was still staring at him. "He's looking at me. Can you see him looking at me?"

"I'm not sure what you mean, darling," I answered.

"His eyes are looking at me." His eyes were closed.

"When you move him, does anything come out his mouth? Is that why his mouth is open? Does he make noises?"

"He can't make noises, love. He's gone."

"But his mouth is open and he's looking at me."

Grief affects us all in different ways. Just as the deceased we looked after responded individually, so did the people who came through our doors to see the shells of the people they loved.

"Do you embalm him? Will you be doing that today while I'm here?"

"No, we don't do that here. This is just where he rests until the next stage of his journey." She had so many questions and she still hadn't taken her eyes off him.

"Where does he go next? What do you mean he'll go on a 'journey?'"

You always had to be so careful with words, and this was what I had been warned about at the start. Some people want euphemisms, they don't want to talk about death and dying and bodies and fridges; others want the bare facts. The idea of a "journey" hadn't worked for this woman.

"I just mean when he goes to the funeral director. That'll be the next stage."

"He's on a trolley, isn't he? Underneath those covers."

"He is. Would you like a cup of tea?" I wondered if tea would help, and it would break the lock she had on his body, her eyes were boring into him.

"No thanks. Will he go on the trolley for his journey? Do you embalm him here? Will that stop him staring at me?"

It went on for over an hour, the same questions in a loop, the same concerns. Finally, with a sigh, she stood up. she hadn't touched him at any point, which I could understand given how white and waxy he was. It must have been quite unnerving for her.

"I'm going now," she told me. "You can do whatever you need to do. Embalm him or whatever."

Truth be told, I was a bit worried about her. "You take care," I told her. "I'm sure he knew he was loved."

"That old bastard? I hope he rots in Hell," she said, as she headed for the door. "I just wish you could have burned him while I was here."

I had no idea what was behind that, but it showed me yet again that you can never make assumptions. As she'd stared at him, as her mind had gone over and over the questions about his journey and the embalming, her mind must have been in a whirl.

I had presumed that she was processing her loss and wanted to know exactly what was going to be done to him but, in hindsight, she was reliving her own private memories of whatever their relationship had been. What had he done to make her react like that? How would she process those things now that he was gone? It was another glimpse into a life that would remain a mystery to me, another scene from a film where I had missed the beginning and was booted out before the ending.

She wasn't the only one to be preoccupied with the idea of embalming – a lot of people thought we did it in the Mortuary. If it does happen, it would be at the funeral director and done by the staff there. But that would only happen nowadays if viewings were going to be going on for weeks and there was a worry the body couldn't be preserved effectively. Another reason would be in the event of an open coffin or if they were to lie for a period in the family home.

Some families who come to visit start to feel very unsure once they are in the Mortuary, even before they get through the door to the viewing area. I did have people who would say they had made the wrong decision as soon as they got there and would leave immediately. That tends to be younger people. There is a temptation to see them for the last time but it's not for everyone. Some simply can't take that step through the door. With younger people, I imagine it's because this might be their first experience of death. They're still removed from it, and they have no idea how they'll react – they might prefer not to find out.

We're so removed from death nowadays and we rarely see dead bodies. As I've said, the same death and the same setting can have completely different looks for different people, as well as elicit different reactions. There are some cases where I know the body has deteriorated a bit and I wish I could tell people it wouldn't be a good idea to see them, but I can't.

There was one woman who looked so horrific she resembled a Munch painting; she had died in utter terror and it was written all over her face. When I got her out, her eyes and mouth were locked open. I knew that her children wanted a viewing and I had no idea how I could tell them it was a really bad idea, given that I can't say one way or the other.

They were in the office waiting to go in, when her daughter asked me, "Does she look peaceful?"

I couldn't imagine any word further from "peaceful" to describe her. I skirted around it by saying, "There are different levels to how people look once they've passed. Sometimes they can seem quite a bit different to how you remember them."

"That sounds fine," the son replied. "We'd expect that a bit."

They didn't sound prepared at all. "I think it might be difficult. Her eyes and mouth have remained open which can be a bit disconcerting. If you want to take some time to think about it, that's absolutely fine."

"No, no, we know she's gone, that we're just looking at her body. We just want to say goodbye." There was nothing I could do really.

I went in with them, knowing what they were about to face and prepared that there would be some reaction. However, as soon as one of the daughters clapped eyes on her, she started screaming.

"God, no! Mum! No!" she was shrieking in shock and, I'm sure, in her mind she was thinking that she was seeing her mother in the moment of death. The son, however, was completely nonplussed. He just tutted. I don't know whether that was directed at his mum, the situation, or his sister – and left. The rest of them were completely freaked out, and the sister who had screamed was still in a terrible state when she left.

People do ask what exactly is under the sheet. We try to make the bodies look cosy and the families like that idea but they also don't want to be duped – some of them try to look under the covers to see. If I'm not there, they would get away with it, but if I am around, I try to stop it. There's nothing to be gained from that, is there?

There was one young woman who had died of a drug overdose. Her little boy, who was only four, had rung 999 and said, "Mummy's dead." When her father came in to see her, his only comment before entering the viewing room was, "I hope she hasn't got those filthy bloody pyjamas on. She was glued to them." She did have them on because, although we dress babies, adults wear what they died in.

If the police know straight away that a postmortem will be needed, then we have to obtain permission from the Coroner's Office for anyone to have access to the body. That's because it needs to be preserved for evidence of what could potentially be an unnatural death. However, it isn't always clear cut.

One woman who was brought to us had no legs. Joan was in her 60s and had been in a terrible accident years before, when a lorry had run into her at a pedestrian crossing. She was an alcoholic and had turned to drink practically from the moment she got home from hospital after it happened. She was found on the bedroom floor of her house where she'd fallen, trying to get to her prosthetics. It was nothing more than a terribly sad accident at the end of a terribly sad life.

Her ex-husband was the only person who wanted to see her. When he came in, he was blaming himself from the off. "I knew this would happen," he told me. "She drank so much and I was never able to control it. She always managed to get it from somewhere." I thought, as usual, there was a lot hidden in that.

Although she had presumably been able to move about to some degree with her prosthetics, perhaps he had also been enabling her? He must have seen the amount she was drinking by the piles of bottles that were littering their house. "They'll all blame me," he wept as he stroked her cheek. "They'll all blame me but I love you so much, Joan. I love you so much."

"Who will blame you?" I asked him, gently. "This wasn't your fault, you could never have predicted it would happen."

"No, but I was at work, and she died alone. She has sisters who have never felt we should be together, even though we were married over 30 years. They've never liked me. They'll say I should have been there, they'll say I should have been watching her."

They actually said something very different. We got a call from the police to say that Joan needed to go for a forensic postmortem, allegations had been made that her ex-husband had battered her and that's how she'd died. It was clearly all made up, very dramatic and an obvious lie, as she had no head wounds that would be consistent with that story. The police had to be seen to act on it though. I just couldn't understand why anyone would do something so cruel at such a sad time, delaying the process of putting her to rest. What I was realising was that much of people's behaviour when someone dies is driven by a desire to rewrite history, alleviate their own guilt and right the wrongs they were too stubborn to deal with in life.

I don't think the rest of the hospital had any idea of the many stories we could tell and how much went on in our little department. We were an isolated bubble in such a big hospital; we were our own little work family. Whilst the rest of the hospital concentrated on saving the living, all our efforts were put into caring for the dead and those they had left behind.

Like any extended family, there were some members who put a smile on your face every time you saw them and some members you'd rather not have anything to do with. The doctors I saw the most of were the ones at the top of their game: consultants, specialists, and A&E staff. They are the ones who tend to be there at the end of life, and I was developing a good rapport with them. They took it all in their stride and had no problem with coming to the Mortuary. However, some of the "street level" staff, the ones who worked on normal wards, seemed to view us as something quite scary. I was also coming across junior doctors who were absolutely terrified when they came to learn how to do paperwork. There seemed to be a bit of a mystique around the department and some of the less qualified ones had, strangely enough, never seen a dead body – which meant they were scared from the get-go.

How others in the hospital feel about the Mortuary is hard to explain; there is some sense of family and community with others but only as a selective circle. We're very much on our own. The Mortuary department is frequently an afterthought, I feel. I guess, in their eyes, we're not saving lives, but I felt very strongly that our care helps ensure that people don't look back on the process and feel they had been neglected. We are the ones exposed to death with every "client" that comes through the door. We are the ones who see disfigured and malformed babies, who see teenagers who have had heart attacks, mothers who have killed themselves, grandparents who have died alone and been lying in their own bodily fluids for months. We see the decomps, the bags filled with body fluids, the homeless, the drug addicts, the alcoholics. We see everything – but we can't save a single person. NHS staff, doctors, nurses, deserve all the credit they get, but care doesn't stop on the wards. If I had a pound for every time a doctor has said that they are unable to attend to complete paperwork because they're "dealing with the living," I'd be very rich indeed.

Moreover, my answer to that is: "What would you like me to say to the family of the person who has died when they ask why they aren't able to lay their loved one to rest? That they are not as important as someone else who is still breathing, that they don't matter as much? That they now have to come last in the pecking order? I love my job but it would be nice to feel like we are all on the same side and pulling together, instead of in different directions sometimes. We all need each other to complete the circle."

A lot of the families do send us things afterwards, sometimes weeks or even months later. Flowers, cards, chocolates. I've seen that with grumpy people, too. When they come to us, their grief shows in many different ways and they can be distant with us. I guess they're just getting through it. They might also be upset because they've had cause to complain about treatment on the ward, or they'd hoped to be there when their loved one died – and they carry that into the Mortuary.

Weeks later, they'll come back and say the loveliest things, bring you flowers and thank you incredibly warmly. But it's not about what they give you. I just think during that process, whoever you're grieving for, it takes time to actually say what we did was nice and made a difference. As much as that department is kind of in a bubble on its own, it clearly does make a difference for people.

You tend to get two types of people when it comes to attitudes towards this line of work. One is of horror – "I don't know how you can possibly deal with that. Ooh, I'd be sick if I had to!" The other is morbid curiosity. It isn't just the grieving, it's the people "on the outside". As soon as someone asks me what I do, I think *Here we go!*

Are they all in bags? Are they in fridges? Do they move once they are dead? Do we sew the eyes and mouth shut?

What's a postmortem like? Are they in the dark? Are they alone? You name it and they want to know – and it's all the stuff I've heard a million times. I should have a factsheet I give out! It's understandable as it's an area that most people don't see, but, sometimes, it can cross the line from morbid curiosity into unhealthy obsession.

Then, for most people, death is about so many practicalities. I started to realise that people were hugely uncomfortable with those practicalities. If I asked whether they had been to a funeral director yet, it was always clear that they went for the first one – there was never any "shopping around." I can see why this would seem a bit crass in some ways, almost as if you're putting a value on the life of the deceased, but I can tell you without a shadow of a doubt that there are huge variations in price and provision.

Obviously, it's not the same as shopping for the best meal deal in various supermarkets but I really wish people would get past their worry about being seen as tight if they do look into it. I know it's the worst time to be setting yourself another task, but it's one of those things where the "seller" sets their own price and knows that no-one will question it because of all the norms we have in this country about the whole process. Even in terms of tailoring it to the needs of the family, it's so important to ask. This is something you might regret forever if it doesn't feel right to you.

I know it's hard in the middle of loss to think of such things, but you don't have to have a religious service conducted by someone who has never known your dad and might even get his name wrong. You don't have to cringe when no-one knows the obligatory hymns that are played for your mum who didn't have a religious bone in her body. You don't all have to wear black when your auntie would have loved her life to be celebrated. Do it for them – but do it for you as well.

When I say, "Please remember, funeral directors are businesses and they are there to make money," I often see a wave of relief flooding over families' faces. Someone has voiced the unspeakable. "I'm sure they'll all do their very best, but you need to make sure you get what you need. Ultimately, it has to be paid for and please don't let anyone make you feel judged." It's so awful to lose someone and then to have to worry about paying for it too. Old people, in particular, often say, "Put me out with the bins." They don't really want fuss, they don't want dozens of bouquets that will rot, or a fortune spent on a fancy coffin. I think it's generally those who are grieving who think that if they spend more, it will show more love – even when it can put themselves in horrendous debt.

In mid-September, we got repeated calls from someone asking if there were any jobs in the Mortuary. We kept saying we had nothing, but he was undeterred. "Are we *entirely* sure it isn't Gareth doing a funny voice?" someone said, but it was definitely another Mortuary obsessive. Shortly after the first couple of calls, whenever anyone collected or delivered a body, there was often a man in the background peering through the barred gates of the loading bay. A little strange to say the least.

That month, we were getting calls from him every couple of days asking about jobs. We did raise it. The office staff were advised to recommend to the caller that he contact some funeral directors for work experience. In other words, trying to be helpful whilst also getting rid of him. But the calls continued.

One day, we were told there was a man in the reception of Bereavement Services, asking to speak to someone from the Mortuary in person. I drew the short straw and went along, expecting to meet with a bereaved family member or someone trying to sell their services. We'd had a few chancers offering complete funeral packages for under £1000, with a free will kit, like it was a Tesco meal deal. (That approach always seemed strange to me, as surely the will kit is a little redundant when you are at the point of needing a funeral?) Anyway, when I arrived in reception, I was greeted by an unassuming, little man with a rucksack who held eye contact for too long from behind his thick specs, to the point of being creepy. When he insisted on a handshake, I felt like my fingers had been caught in a vice.

"Pleased to meet you, pleased to meet you," he kept saying, not letting my hand go. "Kenneth Barclay – and you are?" I told him my name and he asked if we could talk privately. I still assumed it was personal and relating to a family member that we were looking after. We sat in the "family room", which is decorated in hues of green with pictures of clouds and angels, and I enquired how I could help. He launched into what must have been a practised and rehearsed script that was a synopsis of his life story.

"Well, now that you ask, Katie, now that you ask . . ."

I was treated to a long – a *very* long tale – of how Kenneth had looked after his sick mother most of his life. He had apparently climbed up the ladder of every job he'd been in and they had all wanted to keep him, such were his talents and people skills (it certainly wasn't his handshake…). Whilst his experience was mostly in supermarket trolley collecting, from what I could gather, his ambition was to work in a Mortuary.

Of course it was.

It finally clicked – I must have been slow that day – that was his head that sometimes poked through the gates when a body was being transferred. I explained that there was something of a pathway he needed to take in order to be qualified to work in that arena, hoping that would be enough.

"Oh no, that won't be necessary," he told me. "I'm more than happy, *more* than happy to do this on a volunteer basis. Just helping you out. My civic duty really."

I was about to suggest visiting a careers advisor or maybe enrolling in a college course when he interjected that he was happy to do nights. "I really wouldn't mind being alone in there," he told me. "I could sleep on the sofa if I got tired – not that I would ever get tired of course."

I explained that wouldn't be necessary or possible as we have an on-call rota of technicians that are experienced and trained in the process.

"I don't mind waiting in the car park and coming to help," was his response. He had an answer for everything – no doubt due to thinking about this an awful lot.

I stood up to leave. "I'm afraid I can't help you, Kenneth. Perhaps you could just keep checking the hospital website for vacancies?"

"You don't get to see the dead bodies with all jobs, though, do you?" was his response. I started walking just a little bit quicker – the last words I heard from Kenneth were, "I bet you get some fat ones, don't you? Really fat women just lying there... I could help with that you know!"

I bet you could Kenneth, I bet you could, I thought as I raced back to the office to warn security. They did well as I never saw his creepy little head poking out during a transfer again!

Gareth wasn't the only person who wanted to be overly close to bodies but really couldn't be allowed. Sometimes loved ones do want to touch the body and can't quite understand that the body itself is actually evidence. It's a brutal fact to get over to a family and all depends on how the death occurred. If the way in which a person died means that the Coroner will be involved (such as suicide), the body itself is in their jurisdiction. They have to give permission to see or touch the body. Nine times out of ten, the bereaved person wants no more than to hold the person's hand to kiss them.

However, sometimes there is no warning about what they'll do in the middle of grief. There was one lady who actually climbed on top of her son who had taken his own life. She was pressing her mouth against him, kissing him over and over, with the trauma of what had happened sending her over the edge. If someone does that, there's nothing you can do other than try and support them and guide them. But there have been lots of cases where I've had to say, "I'm really sorry but the Coroner requires that you don't touch at this stage. There might be an opportunity once the case is finished and the funeral director collects your loved one, though."

It's important they know there might be that opportunity down the line, but when they are faced with seeing somebody for the first time since they lost them, human instinct is to want to touch them and stroke their hair. And you have to stop them. I was finding that people mostly wanted to stroke the face and, if it's a young person, I find that really hard because they're mums. I can relate to that as a mother. Imagine telling someone not to touch their own child who they've brought into the world? It's horrendous to see the looks on their faces. I've put my arms around them and held them, feeling the depth of their pain. These are people who are so angry and why wouldn't they be?

They often say, "Don't tell me what to do, I've just lost my child."

All I can reply is, "I'm so sorry but I'm afraid if you can't manage not to touch them, we'll have to ask you to leave." With the lady who jumped on her son, she was pulling him and clawing at him. It wasn't respectful and, sadly, we did have to ask her to stop. She clearly needed more support, it wasn't benefitting her in any way.

Chapter 5
September 2019

One of the cases I'll never forget was an old woman called Nora, whose husband of over 60 years had died on the ward. Duncan was on end-of-life care, so she knew he was dying, but for everyone with a loved one in that situation, the hope is always that they'll slip away peacefully. Nora had been in to visit Duncan that evening and he was clearly close to passing. She'd said goodbye to him and went home.

Early the next morning, she got the heart-wrenching call from the ward to say that Duncan had died. That was never going to be easy, but the manner in which it had happened was truly horrific. I can only assume that, because he was so close to the end, the ward staff didn't do frequent checks. By the time they had looked in on him, he had "faecally vomited, aspirated and died". That terminology hides what most people reading this probably suspect – he'd choked on his own shit as it came up his throat from his bowels.

When someone from the ward called Nora to let her know, they actually told her about the faecal vomiting. They gave her the most likely scenario that he'd aspirated, gone into septic shock and then died. Then, they said, "If you want to see him, best come now." Nora was nearly 90 and had to wait for someone to come and take her to the hospital.

When someone dies on the ward, they usually lie there for several hours before a porter takes them to the Mortuary, so that part wasn't unusual. By the time Nora got there, two hours after the call, the vomit had started to congeal. No-one had bothered to move Duncan from his bed, and his poor widow was faced with that as her last sight of him. She said her goodbyes, was given his property and left.

When I read the notes, I could hardly believe it. The picture that was being painted was horrific. She wasn't coming in to see Duncan (no wonder, after her last viewing on the ward), but I contacted her to see if she had any concerns. Had that been me, I can't imagine how I would have reacted, but it wouldn't have been pretty. The notes said she had been, "a little distressed, especially as his false teeth had come out with the force of the vomiting." I expected her to make a formal complaint. I wouldn't have blamed her.

Instead, she was the sweetest, most gentle old lady who kept thanking me over and over again for checking up on her. I wanted to go round her house and just give her a cuddle.

I said, "I am so sorry, so very sorry that was your experience, Nora. I can't imagine what it was like for you."

"Don't you worry love," she said. "I had a chuckle actually – I always said he talked shit."

She blew me away with her attitude. She went on to say Duncan had been suffering and, in a way, she was glad it was all over.

"He's at peace now," I said, falling back on all the conciliatory things we say every day in the Mortuary.

"Never mind him, I couldn't bend down to put his socks on any more!" she laughed.

She was just amazing and she made me think that we definitely need to approach death in whatever way that fits best for us on a personal level. There's no-one size fits all. Sometimes, where the relationship has been really solid, it can be easier for people to remember the humour and find comfort in things. Older people are more likely to do that –the elderly are actually not so staid as younger people about discussing uncomfortable things. There's a sense, the older you get, that death is inevitable, anyway. Older people do seem to accept it more and, because of their age, they've often suffered awful things during their life and they've certainly lost people.

Death is selfish – it's the people who are left behind who deal with it and live with it. People find it so hard to come to terms with the things that have happened prior to death. "Three years ago, I didn't visit him on New Year's Day," people will say, or "We had words six months ago." It's all these little things that people dwell on and want to erase or rewrite. They beat themselves up about them. But, actually, do you know what? It's often clear the departed were very much loved and they had normal relationships in normal lives. Those who are left behind, though, often want every single, enduring memory to be a positive one. Unfortunately, life isn't like that.

There are some families who do it better than others – and, I found, some cultures, too. I'd already discovered quite early on about expedited deaths when the family was Muslim and wanted a Muslim death. They were also called "faith deaths." Everyone involved strives to expedite the process, as part of their faith's requirements is to take the deceased as soon as possible after death – so that they can spend time with them, cleanse the body and bury them as swiftly. It all happens very quickly, and the family really come together.

Whilst death often brings about family conflict, I was finding this rare with Muslim families. Their bond, collective grief and support for each other was evident. The involvement with the body and speed of burial also seemed to help them come to terms with their loss and give them closure, in a way that often doesn't seem to happen in other cultures. The Muslim families I saw, focused on paying their respects and laying the deceased to rest quickly. They weren't precious about the finer details, such as how they will be transported and certainly didn't care about what other people would think. This was because everyone in their community thought and did the same thing with death.

There was comfort and a knowingness about what to do that made the process quite straightforward. I'd already known several families in this situation to offer to transport the deceased themselves in a van and take them to the mosque. They lined the exit when the body was removed and often asked if they could come into the Mortuary and help, sometimes just bringing their own van. This was in no way meant disrespectfully − it was just another way of them being involved in the process and being closer to the person they had lost.

When one old woman came in, I was amazed by her date of birth on the notes as she was 108! It was incredible to think of how much she must have seen, living through more than a century. It was an expedited, faith death and she was with us just a couple of hours after dying on the ward. I called the father as soon as I could. They were absolutely inconsolable. If someone is 30 or 40 or 50, you know it'll be exceptionally difficult because, if it's a sudden or unpredicted death, the family probably haven't thought they will lose the person. But at 108, you must be aware it could happen any day. Not for this family.

The man on the end of the phone, who told me he was her grandson, kept wailing, "She was taken too soon! She was taken too soon!" He must have passed me onto four or five other men, all of whom said the same thing! If she had been hit by a car in her 20s, they would have had the same reaction. They were so unprepared for losing her. Or maybe she was that old, they thought she was never going to go. They were so shocked and I was shocked about how shocked they were!

I don't want to give platitudes such as *She had a good innings*, but she had. I know people are living longer but, bloody hell, this couldn't be seen as "taken too soon" at all! Their loved one had experienced quite a natural death, she hadn't really suffered, she'd slipped away in hospital. One of the men did acknowledge how surprising their reaction was, to be fair. "I bet you think this is silly but there was nothing wrong with her!"

It was true that she didn't have a prevailing illness but she had just given up. Her organs were old and she had, basically, been alive for as long as she could manage. However, what they particularly didn't like was that the doctor had put "frailty of old age" as the cause of death.

"She wasn't frail, she wasn't frail at all," they kept saying. Of course she *was* frail.

"I totally understand what you are saying and I appreciate you know her better than anybody else," I told them. "But what medical professionals would say is that putting that as a cause is more than reasonable. You're only allowed to apply frailty of old age to anyone who is over the age of 80, otherwise you have qualify that as to why they are frail, as it isn't a natural progression. But with someone who is 108, I'm afraid they would say it's more than reasonable."

They were really affronted by that, as they saw it as an accusation levelled at their loved one. Within minutes of putting the phone down, there was another son calling, sobbing, he couldn't breathe, and was screaming again about the unfairness of it all, about how she wasn't ready to go. I'd had less dramatic responses to suicides or children dying.

I think she had been the hub of the family and it was just their shock talking. Frail or not, though, I kept thinking they must have known it would happen soon. They wanted a Muslim burial as quickly as possible but they were ringing incessantly and wailing. There were times they were calling but couldn't even speak. They were basically ringing to say they were too upset to ring but then asking, "How quickly can you sort things out?"

"We have to have a conversation," I kept telling them. "I have to go through things with you so that you can make your arrangements."

"She wasn't frail! It can't be that as cause of death."

"OK. So what we need to do is agree upon a cause of death that you're going to find acceptable that is also going to be accurate."

I had eight calls that day with different members of the family; it always went the same way.

"I'm X, I'm her..." Grandson, son, or other relative.

"How can I help?"

"Well, we need this done quickly."

"I know – and I do respect your faith and we are doing all we can, but we need to decide on cause of death."

"Well, she wasn't frail, I can tell you that."

"I do need to just clarify things, though."

"She wasn't frail."

"That is definitely the message I'm getting…"

I had to keep trying to break down and differentiate the meaning of "frailty" to them and to us – and that it didn't necessarily mean she was a little old lady who couldn't move. She could still have been mobile and doing things, she was lucky in that respect. I understood what they meant and to them she was still this incredibly strong character. It was an offensive description for them, they didn't want her to be associated with such a word.

She had gone into hospital after a fall and, she hadn't broken anything, so they thought she was going in just to be checked over. They were anxious she would be persuaded to go into a home, but they had never considered she might die. They had been solely focused on keeping her out of a care home. She'd never had a fall before, even at that age. All the doctors saw was that her stats were a bit low and they did some checks. Then she just slipped away… The family couldn't fathom it at all.

What doctors say about the cause of death has to be accurate – but sometimes families don't want that. However, a family needs to be aware that if they don't accept the cause of death, then it often means that a postmortem will have to be carried out.

That's where we'd be heading with this 108-year-old lady, if the family didn't accept matters. The family both did and didn't have an awareness that their lack of willingness to accept the cause of death was preventing the process from being expedited. At one point, I said to the grandson, "The only way I can do this any quicker is to get off the phone to you. This is my eighth call with your family today. All of them have said, do you know we're Muslim, do you know she wasn't frail, do you know we need the body quickly? I do know all that and I'm trying my best, but I need to be left alone to get on with it for you. I can't move forward with things like this. If you really feel very strongly about this, we can ask the Coroner to have a look but that will delay things and we'll probably need to go to postmortem as the next step."

Muslim families usually say they want the burial to be within 24 hours – something born from practicality originally, due to heat and deterioration of the body. Over time, that has been incorporated into the religion's requirements, supported by the teachings of Islam. Other religions, such as Judaism, have similar teachings, commanding that the deceased is buried without delay. This is due to the fact that the soul is believed to have departed the body, and the body begins to decay and change. The sooner the person is buried, the purer the spirit.

In this case, they wanted to bury her on the Friday as that is the most holy day in Islam. It would, they said, be deemed an honour to bury her then.

It finally did go through. Though frailty of old age was on the death certificate, it was listed as a contributing factor; the main factor we all agreed on was multi-organ failure. I should add here, everyone has that when they die, just as everyone has cardiac arrest.

Part of my job was finding different ways of phrasing things that a family would find acceptable but that are still accurate. For example, if someone has a brain aneurysm then they will ultimately have multi-organ failure because one triggers the other... but they have actually died because of the aneurysm. This woman had died because everything was so worn out and frail. She'd had a shock when she had the fall, and it all came from that. Would she still have died had she not fallen? That was the question I asked the doctors.

"Yes, she would," they said, looking at me as if I was crackers. "She was 108 Kate – she wasn't going to live until she was 200, was she?"

"I just need to know that what I said to the family was right, it's preying on my mind – did she have any underlying conditions or was it just that?"

"No, she'd had the fall. All we can say was she went when she was ready to go."

They found that more acceptable than the word "frail", which they saw as a judgement of this matriarch who had been the head of their family for such a long time.

The funeral director came for her with 12 men from her family in the end. Even the Muslim funeral directors have a van rather than a hearse, it's all very unceremonious. For me, seeing it done so quickly (even with the dozens of phone calls), made me witness the value of that approach. It does mean the family can move on quite quickly in a lot of cases. We have bodies that people haven't been able to face dealing with for six months – they can't move on, and I felt that it must always be in the back of their mind. With that Muslim family, they were still distraught, there was a lot of crying and wailing, but when I checked in ten days later, they were very upbeat and positive.

So many people will go for all the pomp and ceremony, oak casket, brass handles, all that gets turned to ash anyway. Muslim families often say, "Wrap her in a sheet, I'll put her in the back of the van and we'll take her away." It's meant with respect and love. When I first encountered a family with that attitude, it shocked me they wanted to take their mum from the Mortuary and shove her in the back of the van. But, when you realise the way they feel about love and family, you appreciate they just want to keep the whole process contained within the people who love that person. It's almost disrespectful for someone else to be involved.

The process can be done quickly – and perhaps this is where the inequality can be seen. I've seen situations in which someone is on the intensive care unit and a consultant might ring to say they anticipate a faith death. They'll say, "I've got X here and my expectation is that he'll die during the night and I'm about to go off shift. The family will want an expedited burial so I'm going to get all the paperwork sorted in advance." All of that would normally take 48-72 hours, but there simply isn't that timescale available with an expedited death.

In truth, I believe that it should be a person-centred approach and the service should be provided to meet the needs of the family. When it comes to it, everyone is in the same boat. I've had people desperate to get it done quickly: they have people coming from other countries to attend the funeral, they're trying to coordinate arrangements, they are utterly grief-stricken, there may even be someone in the remaining family who is terminal – and those expedited measures aren't put in place for them.

I just think that it should have nothing to do with race or religion. I think that we should be doing what we can for families or people as individuals. If you're going to provide a service, make it equal. I find myself saying, "It's not an instant process, it takes time," but I know that when it has to be done, it can be done.

If it's a faith death and if there is any ambiguity about whether a postmortem will be needed, it will be avoided if possible. They try that little bit harder to get clarity. The Coroner's favourite saying is *On the balance of probabilities,* as you don't have to be 100per cent about the cause of death and, in these cases, they certainly work towards that. If the deceased is over 65 or so, then the Coroner would be very reluctant to go to postmortem unless they had been perfectly fit and healthy, and had died suddenly. The Coroner wouldn't want to add to the family's grief at not having an expedited process. Everyone clicks in like a machine and those families tend to have discussed every aspect.

There are also universal elements – there is a blanket *This is how it's done* approach. Everybody gets buried, everybody gets wrapped in the sheet. It works. When somebody dies, everything is done so smoothly, even if they're repatriated. There's a service here, then they're repatriated within 48 hours. Everything else does seem to be smoother, though, as there is no real question about where to have the funeral or the wake. The men tend to do everything – the women pay their respects but the men take over, certainly with the cases I've seen. It's so important to look at how other cultures grieve. Everyone can learn things from other people, everyone.

Some other people attempt to use religion and people's fear of appearing ignorant or unsympathetic to their advantage. They think if they say certain phrases or words, everything will fall into line with their demands.

In September, I had a man who had lost his brother and who spoke on the phone with all guns blazing.

"I'd just like you to know that I am a Section Leader with the Brotherhood of the Righteous Trinity," he told me. I'd never heard of it – he'd have got more recognition from me if he'd said Hogwarts. "We like to bury our dead very quickly and we know you can do it if you have dark skin, so I hope you will respect our wishes too." This was before I'd even said "Hello" or "Very sorry for your loss."

"We'll do our best to do it as quickly as possible," I said.

"Well, you do it for Muslims, don't you?"

I wasn't getting into that. "We do every case as quickly as we can."

"I've heard *exactly* which people you do it quickly for. The Brotherhood of the Righteous Trinity expects just that same degree of attention and respect."

It was bizarre. If anyone says, "We'd just like to try and move on as quickly as possible," we'd do all we can. But approaching it like he did means – and gets – absolutely nothing. The Brotherhood of the Righteous Trinity needed to work on their people skills.

My experience of different groups and cultures left lasting impressions – but in much more positive ways than the man from the Brotherhood left me with. I found that Irish families really did approach death in a very positive way and they were also consistent in their approach. I really do sound like I'm applying terribly broad strokes to people here, but when you see the numbers of people we do, it's a natural thing to do, actually.

There are always outliers but I found that, even in the worst situation, no matter how they've lost somebody, Irish people would find the humour in it and make it into a more constructive situation. They share stories, mostly funny ones, and seem to really celebrate their lost ones if they've had a good relationship.

The prevailing thing with so many people is guilt, no matter how they've lost somebody. If they've had a lot of input into someone's life, they've cared for them or whatever they've done or feel like, there is often a sense that they should have done more. If they've done nothing – they've been estranged, perhaps, which is often the case

– or maybe normal life has taken over and they saw them once every six months, then they really struggle and try to rewrite history, so they don't feel guilt.

It's not for me to judge what is the best way, but it seems like the most well-balanced families can find the humour in things, especially when people have been together a long time. Those are the ones that surprised me more in the early months, as they were different; when they wanted to share funny stories, it was lovely. I had one lady who was on the phone for an hour-and-a-half just telling me about her mum, and every story had a punchline. It was lovely and I ended up feeling that I really knew both of them. That's a gorgeous way to be remembered.

In September, I had one experience that was far from heart-warming. In fact, it was one of the worst situations I'd come across so far – and still is to this day. An old lady in her 80s had died on the ward and she left behind no family. The next door neighbour was her power of attorney, purely for her welfare – not for her finances, as that is a totally different thing. If the lady had needed an operation, then he had the authority to say it was in her best interest and things like that.

When he called, his very first words were all about him, clearly trying to assert some sort of dominance.

"You're speaking with Charles Tonsett," he informed me. "I'm Head of Logistics at Reed and Mansell. You'll know of them of course. To whom am I speaking?"

I'd never heard of him or his company, had no idea what he would be doing as head of logistics there, and was clueless as to why all of that mattered. I gave him my name – he informed me he was writing it down and taking notes throughout. Everything so far was irrelevant but I let him go on, as to me, at that stage, he was someone who was grieving and that comes out in different ways.

"Now, as you will know, I have power of attorney for Miss Lucinda Ferrier. I assume you are aware of these matters?" I told him I was. "As Head of Logistics at Reed and Mansell, I have a detailed knowledge of many, many things. Now, I'd be grateful if you could give me the details of Miss Ferrier's KL43 tests, as well as her bone density on death."

I had never heard of these tests and her bone density was nothing to do with anything – no-one would have known that. Patiently, I explained this. "I don't know whether you are being obstructive or ignorant," he replied. "Kindly pass me on to the Head of Death Enquiries and tell him who I am." Again, something made up – now he was annoying me. He continued to make bizarre requests, throwing incorrect medical terminology at me and just not making any sense at all. He was being so aggressive, obviously annoyed that he was speaking to a mere woman, but I couldn't quite pinpoint what his issue was.

"You see, although Miss Ferrier was an elderly lady and rather poorly, there were no indications she was about to die. You do know that?"

"I only know what is in the notes, Mr Tonsett."

"Yes, that's becoming abundantly clear," he sneered. "If I had known she was going to die, other matters would have been arranged. There was *no* indication she would die, none at all."

He was acting like I'd put a pillow over her face. "I'm very sorry this has all come as such as shock to you."

"A shock? Well, yes, it's a shock because matters had not been finalised. They need to be addressed now. Please arrange for someone to contact me to further this. It's not right, you know. When Miss Ferrier was admitted, there was no indication she was going to die. They dosed her up on that ward, they kept making her go to sleep."

He wasn't going to let this go. "It can often be a really difficult line between making someone comfortable enough not to be in pain and allowing them to be lucid," I told him, and that was true. It's an ongoing battle. Families want those last moments of clarity with their loved ones but, when they start feeling pain, they have to be helped by the medical professionals.

"I simply do not think you understand," he puffed. With that, he put the phone down.

"God Wendy, you dodged a bullet there," I sighed. The phone rang almost instantly and I thought it would be him again, but it was Stacey, one of the ward clerks.

"I'm just warning you, Kate," she said, "you'll be getting a call from a Mr Tonsett. He'll start by telling you he's Head of Logistics somewhere or other, then he'll bang on about 'matters' needing to be sorted."

"You're too late, Stacey – I've already had the pleasure."

When I got the notes later that day, I sat reading them with my mouth open. Mr Charles Tonsett was quite the character and, the more I read, the clearer his issues became. As he'd told me in his lengthy tirade (I'd be adding another ten chapters if I wrote it all down), he had power of attorney but not executive status as Miss Ferrier hadn't made a will. When he got a phone call to say that the ward staff felt she was approaching the end of her life, he had turned up at the hospital with a solicitor, and physically put the pen in the old lady's hand. He had literally forced the pen between her fingers and the solicitor was guiding her hand to sign a will that would hand everything over to Charles Tonsett.

It was awful – I expected Hercule Poirot to turn up any second and grab the notes off me as evidence. A nurse had come in and said, "That's not happening, she doesn't have the capacity to sign or know what she's doing!" The notes also said Miss Ferrier appeared to be in agony and needed to get more pain relief. When she was given this, Tonsett was shouting at the nurse saying, "No, don't do that or she'll go to sleep! She'll never be awake enough to sign the paperwork – she doesn't need more medication, she's fine!" All of this was documented in the ward notes.

The nurse didn't believe the solicitor was real, and neither did I at first, but she'd actually left her business card with the ward staff and it was in the notes! She and Tonsett were adamant that, as soon as Miss Ferrier woke up, they should be called – and left about six different contact numbers. He was adamant that she was to get no more pain relief nor sedation and that, no matter if it was three o'clock in the morning, he wanted to be there as soon as she woke up. Basically, he only needed her awake long enough to sign.

We did a safeguarding check and nothing came back. I mentioned it to someone above me, told her what was happening and that I was quite concerned that he could fraudulently document anything as he had gone to those lengths already. I wanted to report it to the Coroner's Office, as then the police there would pick it up as financial abuse and if he did try and do anything down the line, it would get picked up.

I submitted a report to say that the cause of death didn't need reporting but that I had concerns. There were two completely different issues; the cause of death was straightforward and didn't need further investigation, but this other financial abuse issue was obviously very worrying – who knows what else he had done? I don't know what happened other than that he kept on trying to speak to us and get information but, fortunately, I had been told not to engage with him.

Just when you think you can't be shocked any more, someone like that comes along. I wish I could have done more. I was haunted by images in my mind of that lonely old woman being manhandled on her deathbed, but that was as far as I could take it. Poor Lucinda, I hope she rested in peace – and I bloody well hope that solicitor was struck off.

Chapter 6
October 2019

There is always sadness in this job, but to get through the day without finding yourself rocking in a corner and needing therapy, you have to see the lighter side of a situation. A lot of them can go one way or the other and, at the start of October, with Stanley, we didn't know how it would land. He was another of our bariatric guests, weighing in at over 30 stone. I placed Stanley's hands peacefully over his extremely large tummy but, as with other bariatric patients, we always had to be careful with the stomach area.

While transporting him and laying him out for the viewing, we'd been able to hear an awful lot of sloshing about. It had become evident that any pressure applied to his stomach would result in the build-up of his bodily fluids violently spewing out of his mouth. We'd already had to do a fair few clean ups and were trying our best to keep him in a decent state.

When Stanley's grief-stricken family arrived, we had to make the usual – tactful – request that they didn't touch any part of him apart from his face and hands. This didn't seem as though it would pose too much of a problem, as generally, family only want to hold a hand or stroke hair, maybe plant a kiss on the forehead or cheek.

He had three daughters, all of them distraught from the moment they walked into the office. One of them asked if she could pull the covers back, as soon as she entered the viewing room.

"Best not," I suggested. "It's better to give your dad a bit of dignity."

"What do you mean?" she asked. "I just want to see him, not look at a big white cloth covering him."

"It's probably best to just give him a little kiss on the cheek," I said. "Maybe talk to him and share a few memories?"

"I want to cuddle him," asserted another daughter. "Are you going to say I can't do that either?"

"As I say, have a hold of his hand, just remember all the things that made him your dad."

"But…" they both interrupted at the same time – only to be interrupted themselves by the third sister who had held back a bit.

"For Christ's sake!" she hissed. "He was a smelly, fat bastard in life, he's a smelly, fat bastard in death. Only time he'd have gone anywhere near you would have been to shove you out of the way if there was a pizza coming."

I was cringing in the corner but almost breathed a sigh of relief – not that there was time. As one sister kicked off at the one who had brought them all down to Earth, the third one launched herself at her father in anguish, throwing herself on his stomach for one last cuddle.

It was almost instantaneous. As she landed on him, it was like displacing the contents of his stomach, all of this green gloop spewed out of his mouth and down one nostril.

"Oh Jesus!" she shrieked. "Have you lot been feeding him PEA SOUP?"

"Oh yeah," commented the daughter who seemed less enamoured with him. "They're well known for feeding corpses in Mortuaries." She couldn't stop laughing, as her sisters stormed out. Looking back at me she said, "Thanks for that. I was dreading this as he was a vile man who wouldn't have given us the steam off his piss – despite how much they deny it – but thinking of him as something out of *The Exorcist* feels like a little bit of karma!"

It had genuinely been nothing to do with me. I'd warned the other two as much as I could, but I was glad someone had got something out of it as I started the clean-up operation!

Community deaths were interesting, too. They were no more or less sad than those which happened in hospital but the backstory was often fascinating. Usually, the patients that die in hospital have got longstanding illnesses or are there as a result of accidents, whereas the community ones include suicide, unnatural and sudden deaths.

One particular weekend callout I attended was to receive the body of a 62-year-old man, found deceased at home. He was found by his wife who had been out shopping. When he didn't reply to her shouts to help carry the bags in, she went upstairs to find him slumped over the desk in the study, wearing just a vest, with his underpants round his ankles. The porn he'd been watching continued on his computer screen. I can only imagine this may have marred his wife's grieving process a little!

Seeing all the different ways that people handled the loss of a loved one was one of the most interesting aspects of dealing with the recently bereaved public. Whilst faith deaths were continuing to show me the different beliefs that people have, I also really enjoyed interacting with Irish mourners (although "enjoyed" might seem a strange word).

One of the most positive experiences I had the privilege of being a part of, was when the head of an exceptionally large, traditional Irish family died suddenly whilst at work. He had collapsed and died, leaving behind ten children and enough extended family to fill Wembley Arena. They booked in for a visit saying there would be "a few of us." Thirty-eight people turned up! The family room has enough chairs for about six and standing room for a couple more, which made it a bit of a squeeze as I went round taking everybody's name and their relationship to the deceased.

"Orla – Uncle Gerry there is my dad's cousin's nephew."

"Jamesie – my great granny was his great auntie. I think."

You get the idea. There were so many of them but that family had such a lovely way of mourning. They went in to see Gerry in small groups so that they could hold his hand and say a few private words. Of course, tears were shed. They were bereft but there was also lots of laughter and love, lots of stories and they sat around his bed, including Gerry in the conversation and reminiscing about happy times and the positive impact he had had on their lives.

It was refreshing to see and I remember thinking that when my own time comes, that's what I would want. Not the sitting around my bed but the love, laughter and positivity that emanated from his entire family which was a joy to watch. They came a few times, in several smaller groups, and they were always hugely grateful that we had accommodated them. On their final visit, they brought flowers and chocolates for staff to say, "Thank you." It's always really humbling when grieving families take the time to do this, at a time when they're already dealing with so much more. It might seem strange to say but I missed that family when they were gone. I knew that Gerry had been given the send-off he would have wanted – there had been so much love in that room as they showed him just how much they cared.

I was still feeling a warm glow from Gerry's family when another Irish visitor came, called Niamh. She was only in her late 40s when she had passed. She had six children, ranging in age from their late teens to early 20s, not much between them all. I swear that you could tell, even in death, that Niamh had been loved. She just looked content.

It's a strange thing but you can see it on some faces even after they die, as much as you can see in others that they have never found true peace. Niamh's family couldn't have been more appreciative of us than if we'd had her lying in a bed being fed grapes. Her eldest daughter, Siobhan, brought us chocolates, biscuits, cake, something every time she visited. And if she didn't come, she sent in a gift with whoever did view Niamh that day. It was almost as if they were visiting her on the ward, they just seemed to take it all in their stride.

They were all so cheerful and upbeat, they'd take it in turns to sit with her, laughing and telling jokes. Usually, people go in and they're silent or sobbing, they come out and have a cup of tea and you comfort and counsel them a bit; but this family didn't want counselling.

"God, she'd tell us what for if we did that!" said Siobhan. "Death's just a part of life, and we have plenty to remember, all good times. She was a brilliant mammy and we're just lucky to have had for her for as long as we did." They just wanted to tell stories and include her in the conversation. It was a beautiful experience. I told Siobhan that and said, "It's been really eye-opening watching you all with her, you have such a lovely way."

Niamh's family were the ones who really got me thinking about everyone's different reactions. I remember when one of the doctors came in, it was like there was a party going on back there. There was, laughing, shrieking, and he asked was happening.

"Oh, it's a viewing," I told him.

"Going well, is it? I take it they weren't keen on the deceased?"

"On the contrary! They adored her – they still do. They're just celebrating her life."

"Bit inappropriate if you ask me," he sniffed.

It really wasn't. If someone was going to visit me when I had gone, I'd much rather they were like that than sat round with the tissues. Every time they left, they would say, "Goodnight, Mum," and tuck her in. After the last viewing, when I put Niamh away, I gave her a little squeeze of the hand and told her what a good mum she'd been to raise kids like that.

Both families were incredibly respectful, unlike those who were still shocking me with their requests to take photos and videos. There are norms in society that we take for granted, such as dancing at weddings and washing your hands after using the toilet. We're still a bit of a way from doing a live reel of a corpse, but I'd say we're definitely getting there...

Before I worked in the Mortuary, it had never occurred to me that anyone would want to have that sort of engagement with someone who was dead. I knew that this wasn't uncommon when people lose a baby or have a stillbirth, in the sense that handprints or footprints would be offered. In those circumstances, such things are often the only tangible reminders the family will have that their loved one ever existed. I completely understand that and think it's by far the right thing to do, given that, in the past, women were cruelly discouraged to even see their stillborn babies or talk about them.

However, I do struggle more to get my head around the idea when it is someone elderly and you have a lifetime of memories, photos, videos and whichever vase you inherited to remind you of the person. When you can remember the good times or look at photos of them smiling in life, why would you want a photo or livestream of them once they had died? It baffles me.

There are no hard and fast rules for this at our hospital or Mortuary, although we do discourage it when it happens. There are no huge signs stating "No Photography", but there aren't any stating "No Music" and "No Dancing", either. I would have thought the "No Photography" one went without saying. However, a surprising number of people seem oblivious to what a lot of us would deem to be a morally and socially unacceptable practice – I have been looked at like I'm kicking puppies when I've had to intervene. Most viewings have to be supervised but we generally use our experience and discretion to ensure that any staff presence is as unobtrusive as possible. That way, people can have the privacy they need when saying goodbye.

On one particular occasion, I'd gone to get a glass of water for a weeping daughter, only to see flashes of light through the glass panel as I approached and her slide her phone hastily into her back pocket when I entered. I let a little time lapse then broached it tactfully, saying that I had forgotten to communicate a few basic rules, one of which being, please don't take any photos.

I was met with a horrified yet innocent expression. "Oh God, we'd never do anything like that! Who does that? Some people are awful, aren't they?" *OK Pinocchio*, I thought. If I hadn't seen it with my own eyes, I would have been almost convinced.

Another time, a deceased gentleman called Martin had two visitors, one of which was his Thai bride. She was accompanied by an older woman, they were both somewhere in their 60s and incredibly rude. They had arrived disgruntled to start with and stormed in as though they were quite entitled to do whatever they wanted, whenever they wanted, and that I was just there to be ordered about.

I'm quite flexible, really, as I do think that grief shows in many different ways and that people can often be so upset that they act in a less than friendly way. But this pair was something else. They proceeded to rearrange furniture and empty their many carrier bags which were full of plastic flowers. They scattered them around the room as if an explosion had gone off in a Crayola factory. Some were put into washed out jam jars around his head (which came from another carrier bag) and they then started to pray with intermittent wailing. *Each to their own*, I thought.

"Would you like a cup of tea?" I asked.

"No. Leave us alone," one of them snapped.

I stepped outside to afford them some privacy. A few minutes passed and the praying and wailing became background noise, as I tried to do a bit of paperwork. It sounded as if there was a TV on somewhere in the distance, but then I heard the noise getting louder and something didn't feel right. I didn't want to intrude, but I also needed to check they were OK.

I popped my head round the door only to find they had set up a little table by the body, had about five phones on it, and were video calling lots of other people! The phones were angled towards the deceased so they could all see him, whilst his wife crouched down to get selfies with him and let the audience see them both together. It wasn't done covertly, and they made no effort to put the phones away when I walked in, although they did look a little sheepish.

"They want to see what he looks like!" exclaimed his wife, as if she'd been showing them his new haircut, whilst a crowd of curious faces frowned at me from the various mobile screens. She seemed most affronted when I told her that they'd have to stop, and she reluctantly put the phones away.

Her companion was a little less agreeable. "Why are you doing this? What gives you the right?" she demanded.

"Well, it's important that we preserve Martin's dignity and privacy. As he isn't able to give his consent, in the absence of a legal document signed prior to death stating that he is happy to be filmed or photographed once dead, we have to assume that we don't have his permission. I'm sure you understand."

She gave me a look I wouldn't want to see too often. "No. No, I don't understand. She's his wife, she *owns* his body now – what gives you the right to say what she can and can't do?"

"It's really not that at all – it's just about his dignity and privacy, and the fact that he can't give consent for this."

"You're power mad. POWER MAD!!!" she told me.

A few more prayers and wails later (though no tears, those had never made an appearance), they left, giving me one final look of disgust as if I'd gate-crashed their party and turned the music off.

As I've said before, the public's curiosity for the dead knows no bounds but, I guess, as my time at the Mortuary went on, I was realising that things which had seemed unusual or prurient to me, were often raised.

Why is their ear, nose, face, various other body part, squashed?

Well, this happens. Just like when we've slept and we wake up with creases on our face or chest or arm. It's the same when someone dies. It depends on where and how they've died but it can range from folded ears that haven't sprung back into place if they happen to have died on their side, to a squished, distorted nose if they've been lying face down.

Why is his mouth open? Why are her eyes staring at me?

This is one of the worst things for families, I think. It's pure roulette but, when I think about the "natural death" of an elderly person who has died in their own bed or in a hospital, there's a 50:50 chance that the eyes or mouth will remain open. Some will, of course, die serenely with the faintest whimsical smile on their lips, that says they are happy to be out of pain and look totally at peace (everyone's favoured option, mine included as long as I have my lippy on). But some gobs will be wide open and some eyes will be slightly peeping. You can never know in advance.

I was getting snapshots of life in amongst death. The ones which stuck with me were where the family really brought their loved one to life. Obviously, any Mortuary in the world will have a higher ratio of elderly people, but when families came in to do a viewing and they said with pride, "Do you know she did this and she did that?" Well, I loved it. I remember one family saying about a little lady with white hair, "What a force she was to be reckoned with" and she had been involved in cracking the Enigma Code.

There was also a young chap who had lost both arms to sepsis. His mum came in and wanted to keep talking about him. He'd opened a charity and been sponsored to run the length of the country as a double amputee. He'd even got an award from the Queen. What an amazing man.

People don't just bring stories, they bring wedding pictures, too. It brings the departed to life for me and I wish I'd met them under different circumstances. I wish I could have sat down with them for an hour and a cup of tea. You get such a strong sense of their character. All those lost stories – and the only reason I'm aware of them is because they're gone. Those families – and more bodies get no visitors than those that do – share so much.

That old lady with the white hair would have been one more elderly fatality, and nothing out of the ordinary, without her family sharing her extraordinary achievements.

The family was terribly upset but they so wanted all the work she had done to be known and recognised. Those are the magical bits for me – the person might have gone but they've had a massive impact.

I'm probably one of the last people the family tell – they will have their family stories, but maybe I'm the last outsider. I do wonder, when is the last time that story will be told? Then that's it, they've left forever. They say, you haven't truly gone until the last person has forgotten your name – and I think that's true. We get war veterans and, I think, you must be one of the last who had survived.

The lady whose husband had died from faecal vomiting told me he'd been in the war, and she'd waited for him. She painted such a picture of them both and was so positive. Those are the highlights, when they bring them to life for me through their memories. It's a cliché, but they do live on in those they leave behind. That all makes an impact, knowing that we give them one more small opportunity to have the deceased acknowledged.

We were very much within a bubble in the Mortuary – almost the underdogs. Healthcare is based so much on what you earn and what your status is (junior doctor, senior nurse, matron, registrar, consultant). We don't earn very much at all and we have no status or hierarchy. Yes, there are different levels of pay and expertise within the profession but we all chip in together. We don't buy into the labels that seem important throughout a lot of hospitals, where staff seem to be defined according to their salary band. They're a Band 4 or a Band 7 or whatever level, as if that should tell you everything you need to know about the person. There are amazing, talented people getting paid very low salaries that don't reflect their abilities and there are highly-paid senior professionals who are overpaid, entitled and show little understanding of respect or money.

Sometimes, there seemed to be a kind of a snobbery amongst some hospital staff, a line down the middle between them and us. A lot of doctors were very supportive and, having worked with us, knew the nature of the work we did and all it entailed. There was recognition from them that we were as much a part of the hospital structure as any other department. There were others, though, who didn't even seem to think we existed, it just didn't occur to them what we did. They would say, *I'm here to save lives, I'm here to deal with the living.* Well, we did that, too. We dealt with the aftermath of the worst possible outcomes, so, when people said something like that, it really pushed my buttons.

Can you get this paperwork done as soon as possible, because I'm dealing with the living?

Can you hurry this up, because I have to get back to the ward and deal with the living?

Can you sort this out, as I have better things to do because I'm dealing with the living?

It did niggle me. Maybe because I was still relatively new, maybe the others were just used to it. I don't treat people according to the title they hold, I do so in response to their behaviour. People earn respect, titles don't. We still had a duty of care – not just to the person who had died but also to the relatives who were unable to arrange a funeral, or to see the deceased because the doctor hadn't finished the paperwork we needed in order to complete everything and release the body.

You get the feeling with some doctors that they almost perceive our input as undermining their professionalism, that we're looking to apportion blame for the fact that the patient didn't survive. There are so many situations where it's clear there's nothing that could have been done, despite everyone's best efforts. But, I think it's a sense they haven't succeeded at what they ultimately set out to do – to save lives. They're pre-empting us and imagine we are saying, *You haven't saved this patient, you've done something wrong,* but, of course, we're not going to say that. We're just trying to do our job, too.

Similarly, there are very clear rules on what gets passed to the Coroner, it has nothing to do with the personal opinions of doctors or patients. It's just the rules and the law of the land. We're in a world they don't experience, and vice versa. I've been on the wards when I've had to go find a doctor and seen the unbelievable pressures they're under. There can be two doctors on a ward of 30 patients or more, call bells going off, alarm bells ringing, patients crashing and so on. It's untenable but they keep going for the best of reasons. It's admirable and explains why attending to people who are already close to the end can come down the pecking order but it doesn't justify things.

Some younger doctors may have never seen a dead body – and the prospect can be daunting. Doctors have to come down and see the body once they had completed the paperwork, to identify it was the correct person and check for pacemakers. I had naively assumed that any doctor, even new ones, would be fine with dead bodies, but there was one who really wasn't.

She was shaking like a leaf as soon as she came in. She was so sweet and so young, only in her mid-20s. "I'm so sorry," she said. "This is all new to me."

"You've never done an identification before?" I asked. "It's really easy, I'll take you through it."

"No… I've… Well, I've never seen a dead body before." She seemed almost embarrassed. "Oh God, even the thought of it."

"Honestly, it'll be fine. You just have to check the numbers on the wristband and make sure it's the right person." I felt extremely sorry for her, she sobbed throughout. They feel things, they're human and they don't have superpowers – they want to do good. No doubt, they eventually get desensitised, but my heart went out to her at that point, as I imagined my own daughter doing the same thing.

"I feel so silly," she kept saying.

She'd worked there for nine months, which was quite a long time to have not seen a dead body, but she was lovely and her caring attitude would stand her in good stead. We're in different worlds to some extent and neither side will ever fully know the extent of what the other does. I suppose doctors never thought about what went on behind our doors, after they'd dealt with the paperwork – and I'd put money on them never thinking that bodies they'd identified could still be there many months later.

"Some bodies are never claimed," Wendy had told me. "After three months, they have to be frozen to stop them deteriorating. If they have open wounds, they deteriorate quite quickly. Usually, we've got a couple of long termers at any one time. That can be because the family is prolonging it; some see burial or cremation as so final, that they don't want to go through it. Or there are some who emotionally procrastinate, saying they'll get it sorted tomorrow. Before you know it, it's been a week, it's been a month, it's been two months."

Barbara had been there for over five months and looked like she was going nowhere. Although she was in the freezer, she was deteriorating. If the family had asked for another viewing, I don't know what we would have done, as she was in a bit of a state.

"Can you give the family a follow-up call?" asked Wendy. "Just check how they're doing, do they need any support and have they made any plans for the funeral yet?"

I'd spoken with families when it hadn't been as long but, with such a long termer, it was likely they were just hoping they'd never have to make the decision and get on with things. I'm always as gentle as I can be.

"I'm so sorry," said Barbara's daughter. "I know we really need to get a move on. Is she OK?"

I wouldn't want to have to define "OK." I was kind of relying on her to realise that time isn't infinite, even for a corpse. Even frozen bodies fall apart. Families tend to think they're being preserved in a freezer. I thought that, too, before I worked in a Mortuary. That they would be fine forever. That's definitely not the case.

"She's fine," I said. "Well, as fine as she can be after all this time. A lot of families do have financial issues – funerals aren't cheap. Can I point you in the direction of some people who could help?"

"Oh no, no," she replied. "That's not a problem at all. In fact, if we pay you, can you keep her longer? How much would that cost, how much is storage?"

That put me in a tricky spot. If she thought it was free, then she might think Barbara could stay forever. I told her that wasn't possible, we weren't a storage facility. I suggested that to give her mother the dignity and respect she deserved, and the closure that she herself must be needing, maybe it was time to say goodbye. I spent a lot of time on the phone with that poor lady. She clearly couldn't bear for the final stage for her mum to be over. But, there is always the worry that they will actually start to imagine what the body is actually like and have nightmares about that. She did finally get things sorted and we said goodbye to Barbara, but it was a hard road for the daughter to walk.

I've also had families ask whether we'll be getting rid of the body, if they don't get on with arrangements. I'm always clear in saying they can stay for as long as they need to but that's quite a bold statement if someone takes it to mean ten years. I think there are people who want someone to take the decision away from them; they just don't want to have to face that final, harsh reality. When they know the person is with us, it's almost an emotional crutch, a form of limbo. They haven't had the funeral yet, so their loved one hasn't gone – they can bury their head in the sand.

On numerous occasions, there have been families who haven't really had a reason not to get things sorted out. I go through the same options with them. Are there any issues we can help with? Family matters? Financial problems? Sometimes it can be something little like, sister A doesn't speak to sister B but sister A really doesn't want the funeral to go ahead without sister B. There's too much pride to say, *Let's put our differences aside and sort out Dad's funeral.*

Family dynamics can get in the way and many people can't put them aside, even at a time like this. We can give practical support. For example, if someone doesn't feel comfortable approaching their sister, we can do that on their behalf. However, if we don't know, we can't help… I would say that for half of the families who delay things, there aren't any issues, they're just trying to put off something that is so final. The funeral is too much for them and they don't think they'll get through it.

When I've lost someone, I've always felt I couldn't really move on until the funeral was out of the way. It brings a sense of finality and forces you to step through the grieving process, whether you like it or not. I can only imagine what people must feel if it's hanging over them for a long time. Most people do want to move swiftly forward. The focus on making arrangements can be a welcome distraction, rather than reliving memories and finding yourself sobbing all day every day. Despite what had happened with Barbara, I tend to find that, for people who are expecting a death or are faced with one of someone much older or poorly for a long time, they do tend to want to move quickly.

However, with a sudden or unexpected death, people can often try really hard to delay that final process of saying goodbye, even if they don't come and see the departed in the Mortuary. The finality of it, of accepting that they won't ever see the person again is too much to bear. So, the suspended state of limbo is preferable. They can pretend they just haven't seen the person for a while, with no funeral taking up space in the brain. It's not that they want a final opportunity to come and see them, and know that after a certain time it won't be possible anyway; really, they're just delaying the inevitable. I can understand that.

After offering support, my next step is to say, "Our concern at the moment, is to give him or her the dignity and respect they deserve. Obviously, they can't be there indeterminately as they will deteriorate. That can't go on for much longer, given the conditions." Hopefully, it introduces an element of reality into the situation for them. Yes, they're out of sight, but actually it's going against everything I'm sure they would want for the person they love. Usually, that's enough. "I didn't think of that," they'll say. And of course, they hadn't – the whole point was to not think much about it at all.

This is why I think we need to talk more openly about death – not just the practical side of things, what we'll wear and who will get your earrings – but the emotional side, too. That sounds like a heavy conversation to have but that's only because we put death in a pushed-away, little box of things that are distasteful to discuss. We don't want to upset anyone about it, we don't even want to raise it. I want to make certain things very clear to my children – I *don't* want to be cared for by them should I become dependent, I *don't* want them seeing me when I die and I *don't* want them feeling guilty about anything. I *do* want them to embrace their own lives and not mourn mine.

Personally, I would choose not to have a service, as the thought of them all gathered in a church being upset is more than I can bear. I would prefer a direct cremation and that they all go and do something nice, sharing, what I would hope are, happy memories. However, having tentatively broached the subject, they're not keen on all of that and feel they'd be cheated out of, what seems to be for them, an important part of the grieving process. I do understand and, ultimately, would want them to go with whatever make it easier for them to go forwards.

The most important thing for me is just that they are kind to each other and stay close. No matter what goes on in their own lives or where they are, they share a bond they'll never have with anyone else and they have to be there for each other. All four of them came from me and are loved beyond words, and that's what needs to be remembered. The best way they can honour my life is to live theirs to the full.

Chapter 7
November 2019

When the doctors offer a cause of death, we discuss it with the family so they are involved in the process and have some understanding of the medical terminology that may be used. We don't want a situation where it's six months later, they're processing the grief, and think, *Hang on, what did they mean systolic failure when he had cancer?* That can happen. It's hard to wade your way through complex information, at a time when you're coming to terms with a loss. Often, people question things afterwards and, because the funeral has already taken place, will be embarrassed or hesitant about phoning up and asking questions. I have never minded at all. I would much rather have a chance to put someone's mind at rest, if at all possible.

The Medical Examiner's Service was implemented in the wake of the infamous Harold Shipman case and the failures in care that happened with the murders which went undiscovered for so long. That service was meant to give transparency for families and make them feel less excluded. Nowadays, the cause of death is always discussed in advance of the registration process so that families know what to expect. Doctors are now required to complete a brief summary of the events leading to the patient's death and state what the proposed cause of death will be. A medical examiner then reviews and scrutinises the patient notes, to see if they reach the same conclusion. All examiners are experienced and impartial clinicians who must have been registered for a minimum of five years of practice. Currently, the service has a mix of examiners that include GPs, anaesthetists, consultants and clinical directors; a vastly experienced and dedicated team committed to improving the whole process for bereaved families.

Medical Examiner Officers are now able to call the family and explain, "This is what the doctors are offering at this stage. Does that fit in with your knowledge of events, does it sound accurate?" Not only does that give them vital input but it can also be invaluable in establishing some history for the patient. It can shed some light on whether there were falls, any lifestyle choices and their mental state, as well as giving the family an opportunity to raise any other concerns. The family can very often give you some helpful background information; if someone has died of, say, an out-of-hospital cardiac arrest after they've collapsed, it might appear it's come from nowhere. But the families might say, "He hadn't been well for a few weeks," which adds more insight.

One of the most difficult issues to address with families is the reason for delays. When someone dies, the summary of death is meant to be received by the Medical Examiner's Office by the end of the next working day. If it isn't received by then, it gets escalated higher up the command chain. This isn't an exact science. For a relatively new service that has only been implemented for a few years, it seems that not everyone has received the same memo, and you can be greeted with vacant expressions when asking for paperwork.

What we'd like to happen is that the last offices are completed and all associated death documentation is finished at the same time. However, staff numbers and demands on time mean that this often doesn't happen – and God forbid someone dies over the weekend, when there will have been some locum doctors or agency staff in place. Likewise, if a patient has attended a few different wards or departments, there can be confusion and delay. They may all try to ping-pong the responsibility between each other – and often take so long arguing about who should do it, that it could have been completed ten times over. It's frustrating for us, and even more so for the families who are relying on the paperwork to be able to register the death and proceed with funeral arrangements.

Across at Rosebud House, bodies are received through-out the day and night, and a bone of contention can be the time of death allocated to someone. It isn't an instant process. For example, with a 9am death, they might be at the Mortuary about 3pm at best; that's after they've been lying on the ward for that time, with a curtain around the bed, awaiting the doctor to verify the death. We know when they've died, as it has been documented. Legally, though, we have to go off the verification time. That's something that families find really hard if the death came late at night. More deaths seem to occur at night, sometimes in the middle of changing shifts, and paperwork can seem contradictory; they know they said goodbye to their dad at 10pm, but the death certificate says 2am. Or, they got a call at 11pm to say their mum had gone, but the certificate says she didn't die until six hours later. What happened? The mind plays terrible tricks when you're grieving. I've had people call me months later – it's been playing on their mind and they can't get past it.

"I'm so sorry to bother you," one woman said. I could hear her trying to keep the tears back.

"It's fine," I told her. "We're here to answer anything, any time."

"Well, it's just that we were at my brother's bed when he passed. I'm so sure that was just before midnight because we got home about 1am, but… oh God, this sounds mad. It sounds really daft…"

"Nothing's daft if it's bothering you," I assured her.

"Well…" she took a big breath. "The death certificate said he died at 3am. That's three hours later. I can't get it out of my mind that he came to, he rallied round for a bit." Her crying became quite panicky. "And if that happened – I wasn't there for him when he died. He died alone."

I explained to her what had happened. Her beloved brother had indeed died when she was there, at his bedside, and the time she thought it had happened was exactly right. But the doctors hadn't got there for three hours, and that's the time they're obliged to record.

"Are you sure?" she kept asking. "Are you absolutely sure?"

"I wouldn't lie to you. I can promise he died with you by his side."

She breathed a sigh of relief. "I've been having nightmares about this. I've been apologising to him every day. Thank you so much."

If I can get anything across to anyone reading this, it would be that you should always get the clarification you need to allow you to move on, to allow you to grieve without there being unresolved questions or worries, especially if someone, somewhere hasn't explained things to you in a way that made sense. I can confidently say that 99 per cent of the issues that families face are centred around communication, or the lack of it. Even when they feel care has been lacking, there are often very real reasons for things that just haven't been communicated effectively to them. It can make all the difference in determining whether someone is able to move forwards or not.

Even a porter collecting bodies takes time in a huge hospital where there are lots of deaths every night. The porters try and take the least populated corridors, but still use normal routes with a concealed trolley. These are like stretcher beds but with a concealment panel over the actual body, so that it looks like the porter could be pushing an empty trolley or have goods on it rather than a person. If you worked at a hospital you'd know, but a lay person would just see a porter pushing a trolley and wouldn't really question it.

The Medical Examiner's Office then get an online notification of the death and (hopefully) a summary of events, at which time we go and physically get the patient notes from the ward in order to review the case. We'd hope to then be phoning the family within a day or two of the death – if it's too soon, they're not in the right headspace to talk. If I see someone has died, especially if in the early hours of the morning, I know the family will have been awake through the night and have to go through all that grief. That's why I'm reticent to call at 11am, when they've just lost someone they have loved, and say, "Can we just go through this?" I know from experience it's probably the last thing they want to do, so I tend to leave it as close to the end of the working day, as possible. That gives them some time to absorb things and start to come to terms with what has happened.

I always say to them, "We've all been in that position ourselves where we've lost somebody. You might get off the phone and not have taken a word of this in. Don't feel embarrassed or judged by that, as it's absolutely normal. If you think, 'I don't understand a word that bloody woman said,' even though I've been explaining things for 20 minutes. It doesn't matter. Just give me a call back and I'll happily go through it all again. It doesn't matter if you have to call back five times." I really stress that as I know it's just awful to be in that void of trying to come to terms with the death, trying to answer questions when your brain is scrambled.

The bereaved get a brochure once someone dies that says, *We're sorry for your loss: here's what happens next.* It usually tells them to contact the Bereavement Office by the next morning after 10am. The information also tells them what to expect. When I phone people, they're usually relieved to be getting some information and guidance on what they should be doing next. They may have already contacted a funeral director as that is the first thing they think of when someone dies.

The assumption often is that the funeral director will do everything. The bereaved frequently assume that there's a domino effect behind the scenes and that everything is taken care of until the funeral, but that isn't the case. Prior to the Covid restrictions, which would come in the following year and change all of our lives beyond belief, the family had to attend the Bereavement Office to collect the certificate. They then took it to the Registrar's Office, which was quite time-intensive and hands-on. When they came in to collect the paperwork, I could see if they weren't coping or answering questions. It was an important interaction.

It was also a moment when I could get an indication of which road their grief would take, in how they would remember the bereaved. Some families are driven to see a celebration of life, rather than the fact they have lost someone. It's not easy to put that into practice but, the ones who do, find it easier.

The other extreme is that negative personalities emerge in grief and family members can start to turn on each other, as old resentments are dragged to the surface. "If they ring, don't give them any information – they weren't bothered when she was alive, so why now?" There can be all kinds of playing top trumps over what level of engagement they had – "I did this, I did that, I was there more than you." "How long is it until the solicitor rings?" "Has she got her jewellery on?" Sadly, money is usually at the bottom of it. One woman turned up with a pot of Vaseline because she wanted the rings off her mum and was in such a hurry to get the job done before her sister got there!

You can laugh at some of it, but other cases hit you deep. I was in the office with Wendy when British Transport Police brought in a mother-of-six who had jumped under a train. This poor woman had been smashed to pieces from the way she'd died and, the awful fact was, she'd been decapitated and her head was hanging off. Her back was missing and the rest was sort of on her chest. It was a terrible, terrible mess. With Wendy, I cleaned up as much as I could without messing up the body even more and she went off for a postmortem. We got her back two weeks later, but I was horrified when I heard that her adult children were coming in for a viewing. There wasn't anything *to* view.

Unfortunately, the powers that be had already said to the kids that it would be fine – I have no idea why, as it wasn't common practice in that sort of situation. When someone has had a postmortem, no matter what state they're in, the technicians and pathologist try their very best to put them back together in one piece and make them presentable. Given that the family won't see the whole body, they'll just see them under the blanket with their head showing, they can be creative – as can we. In fact, even if someone is decapitated, very often we can just balance the head on something. It sounds horrific (and it is), but the appearance of them being viewable gives peace of mind to the family, and that outweighs the rest.

In this instance, we'd got the lady just hours after she was found on the rail tracks. She'd gone for a postmortem and returned to us two weeks later. Obviously, bodies deteriorate, but the speed of that can depend on how they died. With this lady, her insides had been exposed, her head had been smashed and they really hadn't been able to improve on that at all. She was pretty much the same as when we'd first seen her, just a bit cleaner. There wasn't much we could do with her. She had no clothes on due to the postmortem, one leg was missing, as was one arm, her head was sort of hanging by a thread onto her chest, with the back of it missing – she was just in a horrendous condition. I spoke to some other people to try and prevent a viewing and get some advice, but the overwhelming response was that if a family was determined, we weren't allowed to refuse. The body is effectively their property. That said, who wants to view a body in that condition?

To cut a long story short, they did come. We didn't want them to, not really as that could cause lifelong trauma, but they knew their rights and that we had to honour the viewing. When they walked in and I saw that the only girl was the age of my own daughter, I wanted to crumble. They just didn't believe it was their mum. This was compounded by the fact that we had decided we could show only one of her hands (she only had one now). We had pulled it out of the double black bag so that they could hold it – obviously, without being able to see her face, they were in denial.

"That isn't my mum," said one of the lads.

"It is," the daughter said, trying to hold him. "You know it is."

He kept pulling away from her and was in complete denial. "THAT could be anyone," he snarled. "THAT could be some drunk that stumbled onto the track, or some hobo that was off his head. THAT is not our mum."

"Would you like to hold her hand?" I asked. "I can let you do that... and it might help?"

"What might help is if you let us see all of her," he replied, "because at this moment, I don't think that's my mum at all."

"I'm really sorry but, the way your mum died has prevented us from preparing her in the way we would have hoped. If you'd all like to hold her hand, if you're comfortable with that, you might get a bit of closure at this awful time and say your goodbyes to her?"

The young woman thanked me and moved forward. "I'd like that," she said. "I'd like to touch her one last time. She had her troubles, you know, but she was still our mum."

They all moved forward at that point, even the lad who was so angry, and Wendy and I went to try and get their mum's hand out. We'd already worried about how we would do it and how we would position her. Even then, the hand was like something out of a horror film. It was bleached white with the skin falling off, even worse than when we had cleaned the poor woman up earlier. I remember saying to Wendy at that point, "We just can't let them see this."

"We've got to," she'd told me. "We've no choice – this is about all that's in any fit state to be seen, when you look at everything else." I just kept looking at it, imagining it was my withered hand and that was my daughter, my sons, standing there, wanting to touch me but also horrified at what might be under the cover. Maybe seeing just one part is worse, as it leaves so much to the imagination. Who knows?

I also had no idea what they had been told. They knew she'd jumped under a train, but did they know the extent of her injuries?

None of them could touch her. "We can't see her face, can we?" asked one of them.

"Not really – I'm so sorry."

"Do you know why that is?" he asked.

God, what could I say? How do you tell someone such a horrific and cruel thing about their own mother? "It's so difficult when there's been a tragic death like your mother's," I ventured. "She did take the impact of the train, I'm afraid. It's always good to focus on the nice memories." He nodded, and I could just see that he knew a little of the horrors lurking under there.

"How is he?" the daughter asked.

"Who?"

"The driver. The train driver. It must have been awful for him." God bless her, she was so lovely to even think of something like that in her own grief.

"You honestly think we're just going to walk out of here with seeing anything but that… thing?" retorted the angry son. "I want to see her. I want to see her face."

"David, just leave it," said his sister. "The lady has already told you, it wouldn't be a good idea."

"I'm not going to lie," I said. "I was here when they brought your mum in. We spent a lot of time just cleaning her up and then we tried to do the best we could with… everything. I'll be honest with you, David. I have boys your age, and the thought of them being in your position and seeing what I saw… it's not something I would advise, really, it's not. I didn't know your mum, but I don't believe she would want you to see her this way."

He looked defeated, as if all the fight had gone out of him. "None of us know what was going on in your mum's head but, what I do know, is that it's totally normal to think a couple of things. You'll be wondering why you weren't enough and why she couldn't stay around for you; and you'll be feeling guilty because you'll be thinking you could have done something. All of that is perfectly normal. I know from my experience that there's nothing you could have done, I truly believe that. Not because I knew your mum, but because I've known so many people in dark places. When they're in those dark places, the normal ways of thinking go out the window. There's nothing that would have been enough to have kept her. She would have believed that as a positive thing, that the people she loved the most would have been better without her."

I didn't know at the time whether I got through to them at all, or whether they were even listening, or whether they just thought, "Oh shut up, you silly cow and piss off." I didn't know what they were thinking at all, because they were just six kids sat there, holding each other, lost. I was just trying to put my thoughts across, and they were only my thoughts. They came from no great place of wisdom, just life experience – but I was just trying to pre-empt anything they might have been feeling and thinking, as well as imagining myself in the same situation.

They agreed not to see her. They did go in and put their hands on the bag which sounds really impersonal, but they knew she was in there. Her belongings were on the top in a little bag, her necklace, watch and her ring. Such small reminders of a life.

The next day, there was a huge bunch of flowers delivered to everyone at the Mortuary and I got a personal email from her daughter. These lovely people had taken the time to write the kindest, most thoughtful email, to say how much I'd helped them, and how everything I'd said made them feel much better in the midst of their devastation. Even feeling pleased about that makes me feel self-indulgent, but it did make me feel quite settled that I'd made the slightest difference to them. If I'd alleviated even the tiniest sliver of pain, I'd be content. Even if I never get a response like that again, I'll still feel like this job's been worthwhile, because that really meant the world to me.

All of the cases, with youngsters who have lost a parent or with babies who have passed, touch me as a mum. I relate to the loss but, also, I can't fathom that level of pain, because, thank God, I've never had to deal with it.

The one case that is constantly in my thoughts is Jenny who had lost her little girl, Sarah. Sarah was a cot death, a beautiful big baby girl who had just gone to sleep one night and never woken up. Cot death is so cruel, so unfathomable and Jenny was, quite naturally, broken. I'd snuggled Sarah up in a beautiful white blanket, swaddled her and had her ready for the visit.

The first thing Jenny did was touch her cheek.

Then she screamed.

She screamed and screamed and screamed.

I went to her and held her in my arms.

"She's so cold, she's so cold! My baby is so cold! Can't you do something?"

"I know, I know. It's a shock, but she's still your little girl. Would you like to hold her?"

"No! NO!" She was hysterical.

You'd think the coldness would be obvious but, in hindsight, grief doesn't make anything obvious. There's cold – and there's cold. You expect them to be cold because they're dead, but to make that connection between your baby and a fridge? Well, how could you?

For us, working there, we get a bit freaked out if the body is warm, we're used to the cold, but this woman had gone to touch her beautiful baby's cheek and faced the reality of what had happened. Sarah would never be warm with life again.

I encouraged her to go sit on a little bench we have and asked if she'd like me to take Sarah out of the big pram.

"Yes, please – but you hold her. I don't want to."

I must have cradled that baby for four or five hours. Jenny sang to her, she looked at her constantly, but she couldn't bear to hold her because she was so cold and rigid. At one point, I swaddled Sarah even more tightly so all Jenny would be holding was blankets if she could manage it. All you could see was her little face but she couldn't do it. I found myself rocking Sarah and stroking her.

I said, "Do you want me to put her down and leave you on your own?"

"No!" her response was instant. "Can you stay?"

Sometimes mums want to dress their babies or change them, sometimes they want to read or sing to them, hold them or not, have them in the basket and look at them. Sarah was in the big pram. Most babies look swamped in there but she didn't. We'd dressed the pram so beautifully and, maybe, thinking about it now, that didn't help. Maybe seeing her in such a natural environment, in a pram with blankets, maybe that exacerbated the shock of her being cold and hard.

Jenny kept apologising.

"You don't have to say that, please don't feel judged. Sometimes it isn't the right decision, but you don't realise until you're in there. There isn't a right and wrong." Either way, people think it is a reflection on them. She just kept saying, "She's so cold, she's so cold." I felt such guilt – I still do. I should have prepared her for that. Even after all those hours we spent with Sarah, she was as cold at the end, as at the start. Once they're gone, there is nothing there internally to heat the body up.

After a few hours, I did say. "All you'll feel is blanket, love." I thought if she could just get that closeness with her baby, it would help. But she never held her, not at any point. I don't think she wanted to talk, she just wanted to look at Sarah.

"If you want me to go and leave her in the pram, just say, or I can just sit here with her."

"I just want to look at her, please stay. Just hold her, I want someone to hold her. I can't. I just can't." I understood that. It was torment for her. At one point, when Wendy was locking up, Jenny said, bless her, "Do you need to go home?"

"I'll be here for as long as you need me, but I do just need to go into the office and sort out a few things, then I'll come back," I told her. "She's really swaddled, you can only see her little nose." I wondered if Jenny would hold her baby while I was in the office, but when I went back, she hadn't moved. Sarah was still in the pram. For the last hour, it was really just me saying, "We have to start to think about putting her away now."

Every time I said it, she asked for five more minutes. I felt like I could touch her pain. I kept thinking, *This time yesterday, she was holding her baby, cuddling her, playing with her, singing to her. And now – this.* A six-month-old little girl. You'd think you'd got her to safety, just a little bit, wouldn't you? And then, in comes Fate with other ideas. Finally, I had to say that we had to put Sarah away and asked again if she wanted to hold her.

"If you go home and change your mind, now that you know what to expect, just come back."

She shook her head. She said thank you so much and just left. She never did come back. I remember going home and I could still feel the weight of Sarah in my arms. The world is so wrong that these things can happen. I felt Jenny had only got pain from it all, I don't believe those hours were anything other than hell for her.

I can definitely relate to parents wanting to know where their children are going to be. As a parent, you always want to know where your child is, are they warm or cold, are they safe? Why would that change when they die?

I've met so many people who are incredibly blunt, although that tends to be with older people.

"She's in the fridge, isn't she?"

"Well, it is a temperature-controlled environment, yes." You try to dress these things up to not sound so brutally harsh.

"It's a fridge, isn't it? Is she on a metal tray?"

"She's wrapped up well," I'll tell them.

Everything they say, I try to see it from their perspective – they're not really asking that, they're maybe wondering, "Is she dignified or lying there with no clothes on?" I try to interpret it but sometimes it's hard to see it as anything other than harsh.

Some people genuinely want all the gory details, for no reason other than they have a fascination with it. Teeth are a big thing, a huge thing.

When you die, if you have false teeth, they drop. Your gums shrink when your blood circulation stops and very often the top teeth drop down. We often get visitors who say before the viewing, "Has she got her teeth in?" If I say she hasn't, they'll invariably respond with, "She wouldn't like that at all – can you sort it out?"

I do that if they want, but you really have to clip them up into place so that they stay in. For some reason, lots of people want to take the teeth home. I really don't understand it at all! There was one old gentleman who had the most beautiful, aged-leather toiletry bag. Inside was an old-fashioned shaving brush, a silver razor and an initialled, cotton handkerchief, clearly all so special to him.

I showed it to his son. "We still have this," I told him. "It all just seems such a nice memento of your dad."

He looked at me as if I had two heads. "We'll just have his teeth, thanks. Dump the rest." I handed over this little plastic dish with ancient falsies in it and just couldn't work out why so many people were obsessed. To get rid of lovely, personal items and keep a set of discoloured gnashers was beyond me!

I guess teeth are very personal. There's a lot of owner-ship there! The things you think will matter least, like teeth and hearing aids, the things that don't make up the essence of people, these are what bereaved family members sometimes latch onto. But the items that are often personal, like a fabric hankie that is initialled and smells of him, they get tossed. The only thing they don't want to get rid of is teeth, hearing aids and jewellery. All the jewellery has to be kept in the safe if not claimed but, if someone says bin a bag, then we do. It's probably the last thing they used but it seems meaningless. They are free and easy with things like that but, God forbid you chuck away someone's false teeth. People will even make special trips to come and get them.

Maybe they're the same people who want to know how quickly the body will decompose. There was one woman who visited her husband for days on end. He was green and smelled terribly by the time she stopped, and she appeared oblivious to it all.

Other people will visit the day after someone dies and ask what will they be like tomorrow? Will they be OK or will they have gone off by then? It's like they're talking about something in the veg section in Tesco. They have this almost grizzly frame of reference that is so off, yet when they are with the body, they're clearly distraught. The process can be surreal for people and, I think they dip in and out of the reality of it and with what they can and can't cope with. I did have a morbid curiosity before working here, but I don't have it about my loved ones, I wouldn't want to know it about them.

Chapter 8
December 2019

Most mortuaries around the country are full in December, but we were particularly busy because we had a lot of long-termers. Although some of those were people whose loved ones couldn't bear to take that final step and arrange the funeral, many others had no families and the coroner hadn't seen fit to release them. The rule was that, after a while, if they are not leaving the Mortuary, they're meant to be frozen... but we only had one working freezer. There were about eight bodies that were getting mouldy and were in a very bad way. Another game of "Dead Body Jenga" was on the cards.

What happens is, when someone dies in hospital, the porters bring them down and put them away in a fridge, writing their names on the correlating card on the door. However, when the fridges start getting full, the porters get really panicky– they're scared of turning up and having nowhere to store the bodies. If it looks like we even have ten spaces left, they start to get anxious.

In the bottom shelf of the fridge, the bodies go from top to bottom in a row of three. It might seem like the bottom row is the most accessible but, actually, it's the least accessible, as for every other tray there's an electronic hoist. You slide the bodies on, then it raises them into their place in the fridge. But with the bottom row, well, the tray there won't go that low. I had to work out how to manoeuvre the bodies, putting them on the bottom shelf without any help from a hoist. Manhandling the weight – the dead weight – was the most physically difficult thing to do in the job. Porters would turn up, look at the doors to see if any were marked blank and, if they only saw some at the bottom which were reserved for emergencies, they would call us out.

I'd been warned it always got worse in December, as there are just more deaths at that time of year. Old people are vulnerable. They fall on the ice and snow and break bones, especially hips. They don't turn the heating up and get cold, or they can't afford to cook as it means using more gas or electricity, or they get every cold and flu strain there is. It's awful, but they just die more easily. We know it's going to happen and we know that the battle to free up fridge space will start. That December, from the start, I couldn't even begin to count how many times I was called out by porters saying that there were no spaces. I knew that there were a few empty slots, but they would have their own ideas.

Wendy had told me they did tend to panic and had a mental inventory of the wards. "We're expecting ten deaths tonight," one of them would say. They would ask the ward staff, "Have you got any expected deaths? How many do you think will go tonight?" claiming that it was to give the Mortuary an idea of what might be happening. We weren't that bothered because, whatever happened, we'd simply have to deal with it.

A lot of the porters were men just coming up to retirement, and they were incredibly dramatic. One of them heard me cough and said, "You'll be in here soon." I laughed, but he was completely serious. "Honestly – I see it all the time. You think it's nothing to worry about, then you're six feet under." They panicked that they would turn up to the Mortuary and have to do some heavy lifting – not that they ever did. The three of us were constantly having to move bodies into spaces on the bottom, because we knew that if the porters got there and those were the only empties, they just wouldn't do anything. They'd only get involved if the hoist was doing the shifting.

It got to the point where we were all there nearly every night in December, moving bodies about before the porters arrived. We'd pull them out, saying, "How big is that one? Can it go somewhere else?" It wasn't meant disrespectfully but we were guessing the weights. "How heavy's this one, can it fit somewhere else?" We were just trying to get more accessibility. Wendy had warned me, but I was still shocked when the porters started calling to say: they hoped we were prepared as there was no way they would even consider bringing someone down later, unless they could be assured no bottom trays were to be filled. We're good but we're not that good. We can't magic up spaces, so the only thing we could do was move them round each day when we got there and each night when we left to go on call. That way, the available spaces weren't on the bottom but further up – as the porters just weren't willing to put them in the bottom spaces.

We were moving people who were in different states and at different stages of decomposition. We could pull one out and there would be pure, unadulterated leakage everywhere. This meant another two hours washing up, putting clean clothing on and disinfecting everything. I don't think there was a night in December when something like that didn't happen. We were running on just three or four spaces at any given time, which is "full to capacity" in those conditions.

And also, we had Father Christmas.

It didn't sound real and nobody believed us. The man was huge, very tall, with long white hair and a straggly white beard. He didn't have a family to claim him. He'd been there for such a long time, in a bariatric fridge because he was so tall and obese. We physically couldn't move him anywhere else. He didn't even have room to put his arms down by his sides in the container, so we had to truss them together with string in order for them to remain in place on top of his body. That might seem a bit disrespectful but life – and death – isn't like in a film, we have to do what we can. People aren't all the same size and they don't all die in the same way. Was it undignified to have to bind his arms together? He just wouldn't have fitted in otherwise. Usually, bodies are covered up with bags, but he was lying on a hospital sheet with nothing on other than a hospital gown around his waist as we were stuck to find something to fit.

We checked on him frequently and had been calling him Father Christmas since he first arrived; it was just a bit more poignant in December. Santa had died. He had been deteriorating for a while – he'd been there since before I started working in the Mortuary – but, in December, it got even worse very quickly. No-one had claimed Father Christmas and it was unlikely they ever would. Estates Research had to be carried out to try and discover who this man was. But he didn't have any records, he had just appeared with no previous medical files or NHS number. All that we got back was that he had no family, he'd never been married and that a hospital cremation was the only option.

We all felt so sorry for him and would say, "I'm just off to see Father Christmas!" We do make an effort for people who have no-one, as it's just so sad. When someone has no next of kin, apart from it being on the records, you're hit by the fact that no-one rings to find out what's going on, nobody phones to ask how they deal with the funeral or register the death – there's nobody to care. The staff go to see these cases a lot and this man really did look like Father Christmas, which meant he pulled on our heartstrings even more.

He'd been found unconscious in his flat by one of his neighbours who'd realised she hadn't seen him for a few days, then brought into A&E. He'd suffered a sudden cardiac arrest and never regained consciousness. They'd tried to resuscitate him but he died. We did joke that no-one would be getting presents that year, but we also chatted to him whenever we had a moment. Sadly, he was deteriorating really quickly after almost a year in the fridge. His face had completely disappeared; it was purged, gone. His eyes, nose, mouth – all of the fluid had come out and his face had rotted away. What an end for anyone.

The Christmas period was the busiest I'd ever seen the Mortuary. It wasn't just the massive death toll of old people during winter, but also those going out to pubs and parties, and getting themselves in situations that escalated because of over-drinking or drug taking. There were also more people taking their own lives, as I guess it's a time of year that brings situations and relationships into sharp focus. There was a surge, and we were almost full to capacity, hence the constant fussing of the porters, on top of everything else.

If someone has died, then the visiting loved ones tend not to be feeling in the Christmas spirit. So, we are not exactly going to be rocking about in Rudolph noses. We do, however, have a few tasteful decorations up in the office and family room, where there are always pictures of angels, clouds, and a few motivational quotes. We're careful. If you lose someone at Christmas, Christmas will be marked forever.

I did feel, for me, that every day of the year resonated. Every day of the year was a day of loss for someone, a day when their life would never be the same again. At some times, I thought I was becoming desensitised. At other times, I felt raw, with the possibility of death everywhere around me. I knew that if I let it seep into my thinking too much, I just wouldn't be able to do the job at all. Nobody would. I'd found a place for myself in the land of the dead, but that didn't mean it was always easy.

Christmas is a strange time of year to be in a Mortuary. Everyone is in good spirits, lots of doctors and consultants come down, they and the visitors give you gifts and they seem to go out of their way to say how they appreciate the work you do. Nevertheless, that whole party atmosphere, with everyone saying how great each other is, can't disguise the environment we're in, and what is happening behind the doors away from the small office area.

I guess what we struggle with is that, in the hospital, staff and patients often have hope. They're striving for a good outcome. No matter how sick they are, there's reassurance that they'll be cared for, that they'll be looked after. When someone comes to us, obviously, all hope has gone. People are in a black hole of grief, they're in a void. That's why I always emphasise that I will talk to their departed loved one; I do go and chat to people in the fridges, I do have a conversation while I'm getting them ready for a viewing – I genuinely do all of that. Is it daft? I don't think so, as I feel it continues the respect they deserve from beginning to end.

When people want to know grisly details – is she cold on the slab, is he naked, do you just leave them all lying there in a room? – I do think that comes from fear. But it puts us in a no-win situation; we can't really reveal everything that goes on behind the scenes. Not because we do terrible things, we honestly don't, but because it will prey on the minds of the bereaved. I just think the most important thing to us is that everybody is as positive as they can be. I just try to address what I can in the best way I can.

Is he going in a bag?
Is he going on a tray?
Is he going in a fridge?

I won't lie to people. I'll say: "Look, we can't pretend this is where anybody wants their loved one to be. All I can say is, we will carry out our work with as much dignity and care as we would want if somebody was treating someone we love. We have to move them sometimes, but it is done with the utmost care and dignity."

The only time I've reeled away from giving information is when women lose babies and ask me such a level of detail that it seems cruel to be blunt about it all. There was one poor woman whose baby was very small – maybe about 16 weeks. She walked into the viewing room but kept her eyes on the floor.

"Just take your time," I told her. "I'll stay here with you as long as you want me to."

"Can I see him?" she asked.

"Yes, of course you can see him, he's just over there."

"No... I mean... can I *see* him? Does he look like something I will be able to see?" I knew what she was asking, but it's so hard to find those words, both in questions and answers. "Is he just a blob?" she finally asked.

He wasn't much more to be honest. "Usually when babies are so little, they're not really formed – but he's in a basket, he's there waiting for you when you're ready."

She was utterly distraught, even before she looked at him. It took hours to get her out of the room. She went to leave and asked me, "You won't put him in a fridge tonight, will you?"

The words were out of my mouth before I even knew they were coming. "I'll make sure he sleeps in the basket tonight." As soon as she left, I was in bits about what I'd just promised. The baby was meant to go back in a bag in the fridge to be collected the next day. Of course he was.

"Oh God," I said to Wendy. "I just promised something and now I feel terrible. I can't believe I just said that."

"Well, we'll work it out," she told me.

And we did. We got permission to keep that little baby in the basket that night and that mattered to me. That's what I mean about giving people the right service. That mother wouldn't have known any different whether he was in a box, a basket or a bag, but I'd promised her. I didn't want to have misled her, she was the one going home without her baby. I just wanted her to have that comfort, which I'm sure some people will see as silly.

It really was heart-rending to see how many babies came through our doors. Pregnancy loss is still, to a large extent, a taboo issue in our society. When a woman becomes pregnant, we don't want to even consider there might be a negative outcome. This is despite one in four pregnancies ending in miscarriage – that's around a quarter of a million a year in the UK.

If a pregnancy ends before 23 weeks, that's considered a miscarriage – and yet of babies who are born alive at 24 weeks or later, and admitted to a neonatal intensive care unit, two thirds will go home. And 98 per cent of babies born at 30 weeks' gestation will survive. I'm by no means suggesting that many won't have a battle ahead but it does go to show that, in terms of the physical size of the babies we have to deal with in the Mortuary, there can be very little difference between them and the premature babies who end up in a neonatal intensive care unit.

In England, around one in every 250 births is a still-birth, with the highest rates being for women of colour. There are many, many baby deaths at any busy hospital and ours is no different. It isn't something that occurs to people generally. They think of mortuaries as somewhere that is full of old people who have lived long and full lives. Sadly, this isn't always the case.

Whilst there are designated Children's Mortuaries in some areas, ours isn't one of them – and we have more than 200 pre-natal or post-breath deaths a year. (These figures are for the death of a baby at any point during pregnancy or full term – that is, they are stillborn or died soon after birth.) It's a topic many shy away from but, I think to acknowledge these losses, we do have to address what many women go through. What we see in the Mortuary varies a great deal: from very early pregnancies, where the remains are really no more than reddish blobs with no face having yet been formed; to the first trimester where they are beginning to form toes and fingers and facial features; to mid- and late-pregnancy where they're often perfectly formed but very tiny, with heads of fine hair and little nails on their fingers and toes; and finally, full term or overdue babies who simply haven't made it due to either some complication during labour or just mother nature playing a cruel twist of fate in deciding that it wasn't their time. Whatever stage someone lost their baby, the pain and grief are equal. So, the Mortuary team has to work extra hard to ensure that what is likely to be the most devastating time in a parent's life, is dealt with in the most respectful and considerate way possible. As a mother of four, of course it affects me, of course it does.

Most parents want to spend time with their lost baby, as is their right. They're dealing with the realisation that all the plans and dreams they had made during the preceding months, have resulted in the biggest heartache imaginable. Of course they don't want to let go or say goodbye. Whether it's an early eight-weeks-into-pregnancy baby, or a full-term stillbirth, their sense of loss is the same. However, how we deal with things for these families has to be adapted accordingly. An early trimester baby is usually around the size of a small hamster. That analogy is in no way meant to be disrespectful but purely to illustrate scales. Imagine putting a baby of those proportions into a cradle or swaddling them in a blanket to be held – they would be completely enveloped, and it just isn't practical.

Hospitals have a sizing system to accommodate all stages of development. We actually use a lot of ice cream tubs – they just happen to be the right size and most useful vessels we have. They allow the tiniest of babies to be accommodated and held by their loved ones, so that the grieving parents can still feel extremely close to their child. There is a dedicated and extremely talented group of retired ladies who spend much of their spare time knitting the most beautiful and intricate items, from blankets (smaller than the average napkin) to little hats and bootees that would be way too small for a child's dolly. These ladies ensure the oval ice cream cartons are covered and transformed into the most beautiful miniature cradles, enhanced with silk and lace. These precious angel babies, often too fragile to be held naturally, are presented to their distraught parents who can then hold their little one looking like they are sleeping peacefully in a tiny cradle.

With any loss comes a huge variety of emotions; this is only natural. One overwhelming feeling from parents who lose children is guilt. They feel it was something they did or didn't do, that they could have acted sooner or done something to prevent it. Mums ask if they did too much, should they have stopped working, should they not have exercised, did they cause it by reaching up into that cupboard, stripping a bed or carrying heavy shopping. As parents, it's our responsibility to protect our children and, when nature takes us out of the equation, it can be so very hard to deal with.

One case that will stay with me from that December is the death of baby Gracie. At six weeks old and thriving, she had gone to sleep and not woken up. Her distraught parents were in a state of disbelief and blaming themselves for not waking up and for not having noticed anything was wrong. She was a beautiful little girl with chubby cheeks, long lashes and pouty lips. She had been born at a healthy 8lb 7oz and had been smiling and cooing with her parents before being put in her cot for the night. At just after 6am, when she would usually wake for a feed, her mum had realised that something wasn't right. CPR had been performed for over an hour, but Gracie had gone.

Her family came to see her just hours after she had passed away. She had been placed in a Moses basket, with her breathing tube still in place – we aren't allowed to remove this until the coroner has authorised it. These poor people also had to endure the added distress of the police going through their house, taking photos of every room, seizing soiled nappies for evidence, removing feeding bottles, checking whether there was food in the fridge and if the laundry was done. They were beyond grief and despair and, what should have been a visit of an hour, took over five hours, with mum being unable to leave the baby and begging her to wake up.

These situations are the most difficult to remain detached from. There can surely be nothing worse. Likewise, if I am facilitating a viewing of someone who is the same age as one of my own children, somehow, it's that little bit harder because you can put yourself in their place. Is Christmas harder when you've lost someone? Like everything, it depends on the individual. It's a date to always remember, when others are being happy. All you feel is a stab in your heart about who has gone. But when you lose a baby or child, is there ever a day when you don't feel that way?

I managed to have my Christmas dinner without being interrupted but, that night, I was called out for three community deaths, all people who had died at home that day. I left my house where my own family was warm and safe, just feeling so blessed. I was going to care for three people who had died on what should be one of the happiest days of the year. That puts things in perspective. All three were old people: one had passed away in a chair at the dinner table, and the other two had eaten their Christmas meal with family, then returned home and died alone.

Christmas would never be the same again for those families. It would always be when their loved one had died and the guilt would be enormous, especially with the two who had died at home. Should we have kept them at our house longer? Should we have made them stay with us overnight? Should we have sat longer when we dropped them off? The truth is, however sad it may feel, old people in those situations go when they're meant to go.

Another elderly lady had died on one of the wards on Christmas Day. It was about 10pm when she died. This lady had pneumonia, one of the many who succumb to that condition in winter. There were no doctors around when Beryl died. That's quite normal. Doctors can't wait by the beds of dying patients but they do respond to crash calls and requests for verification of deaths. Older people are likely to have a DNAR (Do Not Attempt Resuscitation) order in place, so that, when they're found to have slipped away, there is no attempt to put them through needless resuscitation attempts that would be futile anyway.

People are often horrified by this but, the truth is, it can take six, seven, eight hours for the death to be verified. They just stay on the ward with the curtain round the bed until there's someone available to do the necessary checks and paperwork. Beryl's death wasn't verified until past midnight which meant that, on all the paperwork, it said Boxing Day. But Boxing Day was also her daughter's birthday and she decided that she didn't want the anniversary of her mum's death to be on her birthday. So, she had to choose between Christmas and her birthday – she picked Christmas because she thought that could be made more of a positive thing when the whole family could remember Beryl, whereas she felt her own birthday would be ruined by association forever.

She actually applied to the Coroner's Office to get special permission to change the time of death on the documentation. I did find that quite strange. I mean, it was correct that Gloria had died on Christmas Day, and it was the verification that took place on Boxing Day, but the reasoning was odd, all about parties and birthday cake... Beryl's daughter was very aggressive about it – the change wasn't just requested, it was demanded and she was really obsessed about it. As I always say, everybody is different. All the paperwork had to be resubmitted because the death certificate was "wrong". If you know somebody's died, you know when they've died, a piece of paper stating otherwise doesn't change it.

We had brothers who died within a few weeks of each other which was very sad. One had got poorly and died, then, very soon afterwards the other died. I remember seeing the name as it was quite unusual. When I saw it on the board, it stuck with me. When I saw it again not long after, with a different first name, I said to Wendy, "That's strange to have that kind of unique name twice."

She said, "It's his brother, Kate."

That must have been so sad for the family. The first one had been unwell for a while, had come into hospital and died, whereas his brother had a very sudden death after chest pains and a heart attack. When it's people who are together, from a family or a couple, we put them in fridges that are adjacent to each other, or above and below. I know that probably seems really silly, but it feels right. It's really sad when you get an old couple. There was one couple that month which really touched me. They had been married for over sixty years when they came to us.

The lady, Janet, had come into hospital and the gentle-man, Hugh, had gone to pieces without her. He ended up in hospital shortly afterwards, as he wasn't coping and had become poorly – he just couldn't function without her. All Hugh wanted, all the time, was to know how his precious Janet was. They were on different wards but the nurses were going back and forth, as both were worried about the other, and they passed messages through the ward staff. It would have broken your heart to read the notes. The nurses were trying to arrange for the couple to see each other, but Janet died. The nurses thought it was going to happen but not quite as quickly as it did. Hugh just went to pieces and died soon after. They were put together, as was another couple where the woman went first and the man went the next day. They didn't even have any family, they'd only ever had each other.

A lot of old couples really struggle, but I think the men do even more. With Hugh and Janet, the family had to deal with burying their mum and their dad. The man who was organising the funeral, their son, had buried his daughter earlier that year. He actually got a lot of comfort that his parents had been together. He was so worried what would have happened to his dad if he'd held on for years, as his parents had never been apart since the day they married.

"Are they in the same room?" he asked. People don't know what the setup is. Some of them think there is a separate room for every person.

"We've laid them next to each other," I told him, but didn't mention fridges or anything like that. They were as close as we could possibly make them. I think it might be a blessing to go that way. If you've been beside someone for almost all your life, then you're left – I can't even imagine what their life would be like.

I had always known that sometimes I cared too much about things but, in the Mortuary, I saw that as a plus. People needed that care, even if they had died – we all need dignity and respect, after all. My own past has been a difficult one. I was sexually abused by my maternal uncle, which was enabled by my mother who was never there for me in any way, shape or form. When people hear that you've got a bit of a tragic background, they often base their opinions of you on that – which I hate. They can go from disliking you to feeling sorry for you in a flash. No thanks – if you don't like me, that's fine! I don't need allowances made and certainly don't need pity. Yes, I had a rubbish childhood, but I've come out the other side and am finally starting to feel comfortable in my own skin. I don't really have any time for disingenuous people who "process" me through the notion that I'm some sort of victim.

In the Mortuary, there was none of that. It was nice to be in an environment where nobody I was dealing with on a day-to-day basis knew anything about my past. I just went in there to see if it was the right place for me, to do the best I could. I did feel that I was contributing in a way that mattered. Maybe it was because we only had "clients" for such a short amount of time. With the hoarders, there was no end. I knew they would just end up needing help again, without any sort of mental health support. Whereas working with the dead was a very specific sort of interaction. Even with the long termers, they wouldn't be there forever, and they didn't judge me anyway. There was a value to be had in actually defining myself *by* myself. Wendy was always supportive but I also had to admit – and this was hard, as I can have very low self-esteem – that I was good at this.

I was learning lessons not just about me, but about the basics of our human existence. I know it sounds cheesy, but the main things I want to impress upon everyone is not to wait for things in life and also to tell people at every opportunity that you love them. Families who lost people at, or close to, Christmas seemed to feel this even more keenly. I don't think I dealt with anyone that month, who lost an elderly parent or relative, who didn't say they wished they had done more, wished they had been there more.

We take others for granted, we really do – and, unless we get out of that habit, we'll be in that position of regret one day. I find that so sad. I've always been tactile but I'm even more open now after seeing many, many visitors who only needed to put their pride to one side and say something. I'm not stubborn any more and I don't hold a grudge, whether it's someone I'm close to or someone that I'm never going to see again. I don't let the small things bother me.

I try to be thankful – for example, when I lose people I love, rather than miss them (although, of course, I do), I try to not focus on the negatives. I'd just say to everyone, have a think about what you're doing. Is it worth it, all the little things we stress about, all the pettiness we fixate on? It's all so meaningless at the end of the day. What does life boil down to? Your relationships and what you leave behind in someone else's mind and heart.

I'm not religious at all – I had Catholicism thrust on me in my childhood by people who were far from virtuous – but that doesn't mean I don't believe in anything. I don't know *what* I believe in, maybe I'm just hedging my bets like lots of people. Part of me thinks when you're gone, you're gone. Your light goes out and you're switched off. There's no consciousness, so what is there to be scared of? We don't fear being asleep or the time before we were born, so surely this is similar? But another part, buried deep, buys into the idea that death could be just another stage of life and that there is something afterwards, whatever that something is. I still don't think it's anything to be scared of.

There's been nothing like that in my job. I haven't been creeped out by anything, at any point. But, like the questions about open mouths and sewn up eyes, I do get a lot of people who want to know: *Have you seen anything? Do you think the place is haunted? Don't you get scared with all those dead bodies at night? Don't you worry they'll do something?* No. No, I don't. For me, with my childhood, the living have always been more of a threat. Demons walk amongst us, they don't come out of Mortuary fridges at midnight – and, even if they did, I'd probably rather sit down and have a cup of tea with them than go through what I'd experienced in the years before I got to this place.

Chapter 9
January 2020

The month before, I'd been poorly, but just thought it was a Christmas flu. There seemed to be a lot of people unwell at that point, especially the hospital staff. The weird thing about this bug, though, was that we'd lost our sense of smell completely. I'd never had anything like that before. I was wiped out, but not being able to smell anything at all was weird.

My son had it, too. We kept checking, waving things under our noses just to make sure.

"What about that?" my son asked, shoving an onion at me.

"Nope. Nothing. You?" I asked.

"Not a thing. This?" he questioned, with a block of cheese under my nostrils.

"You'd be as well waving fresh air at me," I replied. "Nothing's getting through at all. Maybe I should go back to some of those hoarder houses – I wouldn't be gagging now!"

It was the strangest thing.

By January 2020, news was starting to trickle through that there were people in China walking around with masks on all the time, because of some new virus. As far as I can remember, it was pretty much dismissed even when we were all warned that this new thing was highly contagious and heading for the UK. Let it come, we thought. Winter was always bad in the Mortuary, with vulnerable people dying at much higher rates. Another cold wouldn't make much difference, we were used to different strains every year. It would all be fine.

Going into January, we were still pretty much full to capacity and the porters continued to be twitchy, especially since none of the long termers had been released by the Coroner over the Christmas period. One night in January – well, morning as it was 2am – I was woken by the on-call phone to say we had a body coming in. When I'd left earlier in the day, there had been around eight spaces left. In the meantime, the porters had delivered four more deceased down from the wards which meant that, on my arrival, there were four spaces left.

When I got there, the porters were already waiting, having wheeled the next deceased person in. They didn't look happy, which wasn't that unusual – actually, maybe they were more perplexed. I pointed out the few spaces that were left on the bottom but, the ensuing sharp intakes of breath and head scratching apparently meant that they weren't prepared to "put their backs out" struggling with those. There was also the fact that the newly deceased resident was just under 20 stone, which was a bit of a workout even for two people. He was also barely at the pearly gates. When they're still in a soft and floppy state, people are harder to move than when they are, shall we say, a little more rigid. I did wonder what the porters expected me to do. I offered to help with moving her but that started the huffing and puffing again.

"You'll have to make some space," was the only pearl of wisdom they could offer. They expected me – alone – to move the same 20 stone body that the two of them together felt unable to do.

"That's going to take a bit of time," I began, but the words were hardly out of my mouth before they'd made a hasty retreat because they suddenly had several important calls waiting for them. They disappeared in a cloud of dust, leaving me in the Mortuary, in the middle of the night, on my lonesome (apart from 350 residents), trying to figure out how I was going to create accessible spaces. It would be another session of Dead Body Jenga, I guessed.

I had to go through all of the fridges trying to identify the smaller bodies that I might be able to move on my own. Appearances can be deceptive with corpses – little old Elsie who looks so frail and tiny on a tray can be a lot heavier than she looks when you come to move her on your own, bearing in mind that everything has to be done with the utmost respect and dignity. I started the body swapping. A fly on the wall observing would have had me sectioned, as I spent the next two hours moving smaller bodies to bottom shelves and freeing up accessible spaces for the porters, whilst all the time talking to whichever deceased I was dealing with and apologising for the disruption. I even said sorry for getting someone's name wrong at one point. I did question myself when I realised I was telling them to go back to sleep as I was done with them and I'd try to be quiet now, but thought I could be excused given the circumstances.

At that point, I was dripping in sweat, even in a refrigerated environment, my back felt like it was breaking, I was sleep deprived and officially due back in work in approximately five hours. Moving the bodies was only half of the problem, I also had to make sure that the names were swapped over on the fridge doors – Elsie's family would get a shock if they decided to have an open casket and discover she'd grown a full beard and developed a bald spot because I forgot to change the name when I moved her, and they had received big, bearded, burly Bob instead. This sort of pressure wasn't something I'd anticipated when I'd applied for the job! I crawled into bed several hours later, practically delirious with exhaustion and convinced that someone, at some point, was going to end up with the wrong body. Luckily, that didn't happen but it wouldn't have surprised me.

Elsie and Bob didn't get muddled up but odd things do happen sometimes. Working in a Mortuary is an emotional business and you need a bit of a dark sense of humour in order to get through the day. That might be interpreted as disrespectful by some, but I think that anyone who works in a similar environment, where they're surrounded by death and sadness, will understand. It's a coping mechanism and a way of keeping everyone's spirits lifted. If you take on board all the emotions involved, you won't be able to function and will be of no help to anyone.

We take the responsibility of looking after people's deceased loved ones very seriously. We always keep our promises and complete requests, despite the fact that no-one would know otherwise if we decided to have a disco in there every night. Requests vary enormously: simply telling them that they're loved and missed; that the family is sorry for their most recent argument or disagreement; giving family updates; covering them up with blankets because they hated the cold; putting teddies, letters and keepsakes in with them; or being asked to stroke their hair or hold their hand. The only requests I haven't fulfilled are when I was asked to kiss someone (which is against health and safety advice, and many more regulations) and asked to dress someone else in lacy lingerie. I said they could discuss this possibility with their funeral director, and quickly changed the subject.

It goes without saying that a stark, chilled, Mortuary isn't an environment that any of us would ever choose for our loved ones. So, we try to put the focus on the fact that all our "residents" are not just names on a door to us, they're patients in our hospital who we'll continue to care for to the very best of our capabilities with dignity and respect. We are always aware that they're loved, missed and being grieved for – if they're one of the lucky ones.

Some things always surprised me, even after working there for a while. You think you've seen everything but you haven't. At the same time, you get on with the job. You don't always get a pat on the back when you go to work. You have to try and do it to the best of your ability and that's it. But, in this job, I did often get nice things said to me and that's not something I'm terribly comfortable with. I kind of felt I'd found my niche I guess, as far as paid employment goes. You can't bring someone back and you are not saving lives, but you're making a bit of a difference in helping people deal with things.

When a young person dies, there is a sense of such tragedy. From what I'd seen, these losses were usually due to suicide or accidents. My first experience of the difference in how generations can approach death really hit me when the body of a teenage lad called Jay was brought into us. His parents and two sisters came to the viewing, and were naturally distraught. Jay had thrown himself off a local bridge and there were quite a few newspaper stories about the tragedy. These stories had all said that no-one had any idea that he was struggling with his mental health, but Jay's mum had a different sense of what had been going on.

"He hadn't been happy for months," she told me, caressing her boy's cheek as she cried. "We had no idea what to do. I did get him to go to our GP and he was waiting to speak to someone. He'd had a referral, but the waiting lists are so long . . ." her voice trailed off.

"They do what they can," her husband said, trying to hold her.

"Well, it's not enough, is it? Or he wouldn't be lying there like that now. I don't know why his friends said they had no idea. So many of them chatted to the journalists and, when I read it all, I just thought, 'How? How could you not know? His arms were covered in scars from where he'd been cutting.' He hadn't been himself for God knows how long. I don't know what started it, but there was obviously something wrong."

They were such a lovely family and they stayed with Jay for an hour or so. As they went to leave, one of his sisters said to me, "Can I take some photos of him?"

My response was the same as always, "We do ask that you don't because it doesn't really respect the dignity of the deceased. They can't give their consent. I'm very sorry."

She looked at her other sister who shrugged. "Told you so."

"But we really need them," said the first girl. "I want to do a crowdfunder for Jay – everyone says they'll donate, and we can set up a charity or something. We really need some pics of Jay to get people to get involved."

Her dad interrupted at that point. "For God's sake, stop it! A bloody charity? What for? He's not even buried yet. Are you and all your mates going to set up a charity for lads whose best pals don't even notice what's going on? It'll be a bloody plaque at the bridge and a load of you pouting for your stupid Insta pages, won't it?"

I did think there was an element of truth to what he said. I'd seen a similar reaction before, although not one as clear cut as this. I think it's a combination of things: that the younger generation do want to go above and beyond, they do want horse drawn carriages, they do want flowers that are enormous, they do want a show because the death is unnatural and it shouldn't have happened at that age. The reality is, if we put on something for our granny, no-one cares. But, for a young person, people want part of the drama and they're happy to put their hand in their pocket. For Mary who is on her pension and has lost her husband of 60 years, well there's no Insta-ready grief for that, is there? No-one really wants to help.

At the opposite end of death and funerals, as social media events, are direct cremations. These are becoming increasingly popular. Most funeral directors now offer them, with some specialising in just those, even advertising that they provide the one type of service for a fixed price. With a direct cremation, the body is just taken from the Mortuary to the crematorium. There is no service and no-one attending to say goodbye as the coffin goes. Everything is done as simply as possible and the family are called to say it's over and they can have the ashes, if they choose to do so. People are almost embarrassed by direct cremations but there is no judgement. They sometimes emphasise that the person wanted it but, it's almost as if they feel it's a reflection of how much they cared for them. It's really not. A horse with plumage doesn't mean you loved someone more.

Some cultures do really push the boat out, though. One funeral director said to me, "Gypsy funerals are like gypsy weddings – they're big and brash and there's no expense spared. I've just had one travelling family spend £40k on a send-off – that'll keep me going for a while." God knows what the mark-up was on an event like that. If someone says they just can't afford it, all we can do is offer a hospital service. Here, the trust applies for funding, once it has been seen that all other avenues have been exhausted.

A lot of people who are dying or know they are going to die, don't want their families to face the expense of a funeral and they don't like the idea of people mourning in a church for them. In our region, we have TV adverts all the time for direct cremations. There's no cost for cars or anything fancy, it's like a shuttle service taking the body from one place to the other in their own private ambulance. It costs about a quarter to a half of the more traditional services, as there is very little to be paid for.

We have definitely seen an increase in hospital funerals being requested. Basically, when a family says that they haven't any way of paying for a funeral, we give them all the avenues they can utilise, such as welfare rights, and advise them, without being intrusive. If someone's income is low or they're on benefits, then the benefits agency will usually help – you won't get a horse-drawn carriage but the basic costs of a cremation will be met.

There were a few things which stayed the same in the middle of all the instability and fear that was caused by

Covid. Traditionally and historically in most of the UK, women tend to carry the burden for a lot of the work surrounding death and this isn't really changing. Women are the ones who are calling and they are the ones trying to make sense of it all. I'd say in 80 per cent of cases, the women take over. They absorb the emotional side of it much more, too. It's quite rare that I will speak to a man and he will get really upset. He might have a broken voice or he'll go quiet, but then he will become swiftly apologetic. "You're upset, please take your time," I'll say. But even in this day and age, it seems it's almost an embarrassment that men act that way, even slightly, so they try to be stoical.

Maybe some of it comes from the time when women would be responsible for the laying out of bodies, organising wakes and making sure that everyone who knew the deceased was contacted. They would deal with family rifts, with the emotions, with every detail right down to making sure everyone was fed and watered during this hard time. A lot of that lingers on. Even when it's someone who isn't directly related, you won't often catch a man leaving a pasta bake on the doorstep of a neighbour, to help them out when they're grieving.

Women are at both ends of life – birth and death. I think they also like to feel a sense of control, as it helps them to feel they're doing something positive and moving the process along. You can't alter the outcome of what's happened, can you? You can't change or improve things, so the only thing you *can* do is make arrangements and try to organise things.

I see a massive difference between widows and widowers. When it's an elderly gentleman who has lost his wife, and they've been together a long time, it's as if the widower has been plucked from the sky and put on an alien planet. They're completely disorientated and lost. Women want to talk about their marriage and what a good husband he's been, joke about the bad times, and tell lots of stories. I'd never yet met a man who had been married for over 40 or 50 years who dealt with it all; they always seemed to pass it on to their daughter, if they had one, or their son, if not. They just can't cope. You can barely hear them, they can't accept what has happened. On more than one occasion, I have seen a surname come up again, not long after a woman passing – and it's the husband, they've followed quickly. It's like they'd just given up. There are exceptions to this, of course, but that was generally what I saw.

Whether it is a straightforward Mortuary-to-funeral director death, the Coroner is involved or there is a postmortem, I always say to people: "When you get off the phone, if there's something you haven't taken in, then please call back – whether that's tomorrow, next week or in six months. If there's ever a query, a concern or something that is playing on your mind, then call us, as we want to make sure you can move forwards as best you are able to." I always hope they take it on board as I genuinely mean it.

Quite often, I have had families who would call and say, "I spoke to you back in February and, I know it's summer now, but I can't stop turning some things over in my mind. I don't know if you remember me, I lost this person…" Sometimes I do recall them instantly but, when you're dealing with so many deaths a day, it can be hard. I can always reorientate myself if they give me enough information, though, and I can usually tell them what they need to know – whether it's something that happened "behind the scenes" or a bit of comfort. They might be thinking about getting a memorial plaque or they could even just want to talk to someone who was involved in the process at that time and has a link to their loved one. As Covid cases grew, there were more and more questions, and I was sure that would go on as long as this virus was taking over our lives and our deaths. People had so much to ask, but, for once, I didn't have the answers. We were in the dark, too.

I came in one morning and Wendy was in a bit of a flap.

"I just need to change these bodies and tags," she said. "The names are so similar – I've got Maisie Evans and Daisy Evans." As she was talking, it filtered through to me that I knew someone called Maisie Evans.

"What? Who's that?" I asked, looking at the board with the names. "Maisie Evans, did you say?"

"Yeah, but they put Daisy on her one, so I have to change it."

"Bloody hell, Wendy… How old is she? I went to school with a Maisie Evans, so I hope she's not my age."

"I think she was actually. I'm getting her out now, anyway."

My heart sank as she uncovered the body. It was indeed Maisie who I'd been to school with. I hadn't known, as I don't use social media, but there had been a lot of posts about a woman jumping from a motorway bridge. Nothing phased me any more: I've seen jumpers we've had to assemble and we've had bodies to put back together so often. But having not seen this girl since we were 15, my heart broke. What on earth had happened to her to bring her to this point?

There's an epidemic of suicide out there and there's very little being done about it. Maisie won't be the last I see who feels she just can't go on.

In terms of practical rather than emotional aspects, the thing I hated most was how people got about money – who will get what (property, cash and so on) and that starts instantly. There are those who are keen to claim, "I loved him more." When the story starts to unravel that they never did anything for him, it turns out they're keen to get his watch. It's always a competition with scenarios like that. I think some people tend to rewrite history, so that they can live with whatever happened and they can feel good about themselves. When you see how vitriolic some people can be, it's awful. When I've lost someone, I haven't had the presence of mind to give a monkey's really. I couldn't care less where their earrings are, but some people go to huge lengths both to get "stuff" and to exclude anyone who they think might try to get the goodies before them. It's nasty minded. Death doesn't change people – that is who they are and nothing will soften them.

There was one case which really made me think that some people just have no shame. A young lad had gone off the rails and had been living rough. He was estranged from his mum and we had to Estates Research to find her. He'd died a drug-related death but she didn't know the story as they hadn't been in touch for a long time. She knew nothing about his life. She wouldn't even have known if it had been a good one and he'd cleaned himself up.

"Are you wanting to take responsibility for the funeral?" I asked her.

"I'm not sure," she replied. "Will I get any money from it?" She was very clear and unapologetic: if there were any assets, she'd do it; but if he didn't have a penny to his name, she wouldn't. That was her child. You bring them into the world and that's your response? She wasn't bothered.

"Has he got anything?" she asked again. "What was in his property log? I might be able to help if there's something there. Is there?"

"If you're on benefits, you can get help with the cost of the funeral. But, really, this is about whether you want to do the funeral at all. If you don't, the hospital will do it."

"But has he got anything? I bet he hasn't. No, I don't think I'll bother."

And that was that. He had nothing and he got nothing, just a hospital funeral. From his own mother. I see the best and the worst in people. I think the best is when, as I've said, people have died in the most horrific circumstances but their loved ones still seem really predisposed to making the best out of their lot in life. That is the best of people, when they can be so forgiving.

Others can be just a bit too involved – or they try to be. Brian definitely fell into that category.

His wife, Kerry, was in her 40s and absolutely covered, I mean *covered*, with tattoos. There was barely an inch of skin that could be seen, a bit like the man whose son had got his dad's face inked the day after he died. Kerry was in her 50s and, as well as tattoos, she'd clearly been a fan of piercings. Her ears were covered in studs and rings, she had them in her belly button, her eyebrows, her lip. She had a bullring through her nose, on her clavicle, through her septum, through her helix and tragus on her ear, everywhere we could see, there was another one.

She was an alcoholic and had died after falling down some stairs when she was heavily drunk. It was unexpected in that she'd fallen, but not unexpected in that she was such a heavy drinker. It would always have been a potential tragedy if she fell in that condition. For her family, though, it probably would have been a shock, even if she was a ticking timebomb. For them, they probably saw her as living her life and making her choices, not thinking every drink, every smoke, was putting her in an early grave.

Brian turned up without an appointment the day after Kerry came to us and asked about the piercings. "I want them all left in her, is that OK? They were part of her personality," he paused. "Except one. Can you get that one for me?"

"What one do you mean?" I asked him.

"It's private," he told me.

"Well, we can't really help then – was it one of her earrings? There are some nice ones there for you to remember her by."

"No, it's *private*," he emphasised. I must have looked blank. He sighed. "It's a private one in a *private place*, if you get what I mean."

"Oh."

"I'll have it now, thanks."

If the nurses don't take jewellery off when the patient dies, then a lot of families are swift to come and collect it from us (I swear some of them try to get there so they can head for Cash Converters straight after). But if it's not done then, the funeral home usually deals with that side of things. Brian wasn't waiting. He wanted me to go in and get that piercing now, and to hand it to him immediately.

"I'm sorry but I can't do that," I told him. I didn't even know Kerry had it. I wouldn't be looking *there* and I certainly wasn't going to disrespect her by going fumbling. It felt very intrusive and there was a very unsavoury element to it.

He didn't look happy at all. Then he shoved a bag for life on the desk and said, "Can you dress her in that then?"

I opened it up – very tentatively – and in it was a black latex playsuit, a mask, some cat ears and fishnet tights. Dear God, Brian. It's rare for us to dress people because if they come to us from hospital wards, they are cleaned up and come down as is. From the community, they're as they are. However, if someone wants to bring an outfit in as it makes them feel better knowing their mum is in her favourite blouse or whatever, we'll do that. But this? No! He must have thought he could do a round trip. Get her dressed up, collect her genital piercing, have a viewing, and head off. I'd bet good money on him wanting to be left alone with her, too.

He wasn't happy. "So, I don't get the special piercing?"

"No."

"And you won't dress her for me?"

"I'm afraid not."

With a death stare, he grabbed the carrier bag and left. We never saw him again. I wonder what the funeral director did? It doesn't bear thinking about!

Chapter 10
February 2020

Things changed so quickly. In January, we were all scoffing about this new virus that was coming our way, it was all very much pie in the sky. Then in February, it became frighteningly clear that we were indeed heading for something awful. The first time we heard of a reported case in Manchester was early that month but it wasn't in our hospital. We were all shocked that it really had come here. Did we believe it would be something that would change all of our lives in the way it did? No, at that stage, absolutely not.

I remember having a conversation with senior consultants and other staff, including the clinical director of the hospital and, although everyone thought it sounded horrible, it was something we would just get through. There was definitely a feeling that it would only affect the very vulnerable who would have died from the cold and the flu in the winter anyway. Every winter, in every hospital, lots of elderly people die just because they are already ill or old. They slip on the ice, they fall in the snow, they get a cold that goes into their lungs and won't shift, they get infections, hypothermia and pneumonia. Some of them are in houses they won't or can't heat and they are susceptible to whatever the flu virus is that year – many of them haven't even managed to get out for the annual flu jab. Numbers definitely go up, until March; we always expect that. There aren't hard and fast rules, but we usually have about five or six deaths a night on average but winter takes that up to nine or ten. This Covid-19 thing would simply be another thing to threaten the vulnerable, but we were used to it at that time of year.

Even after that Manchester case in February, we didn't have meetings about it. It was just chit chat when people popped into the Mortuary or we were up on the wards. Everyone I spoke to about it, said the same things: *It's the media; that person had been to China anyway; it will only affect the vulnerable who would have died anyway; it's hysteria.* There genuinely wasn't a worry, there wasn't a fear of what was coming.

I remember asking one doctor, "Is this really going to be a thing?"

He furrowed his brow and shook his head. "No, probably not. It'll blow over I reckon."

Towards the end of February, we had a few cases ourselves – but we didn't know. It was only a few weeks later that we realised Covid had arrived. The patients had all been admitted with different things and, because we had no experience of this new virus, it threw us all. People were coming in with respiratory problems but it didn't follow the usual pattern of pneumonitis, which is inflammation of the lung tissue. When someone has pneumonia, X-rays show a consolidation on the lung, but with Covid, there wasn't a huge shadow at all. It actually looked like a cobweb.

The X-rays showed really intricate, defined patterns, something no-one had seen before. Doctors had no idea what these patterns were. They couldn't explain them and were getting second opinions. They said it was some kind of pneumonia but they weren't sure what variant. The consensus was basically, *What the hell is it?* The overriding factor was that respiratory systems closed down. Patients needed more and more oxygen just to function, just to breathe, until eventually they died. At that point, the victims were older people who you could technically say had co-morbidities, or patients who were obese. Later, we would understand these are massive factors but, at that stage, it was easy to blame what was happening on them being elderly or overweight. The virus was sneaking in.

Life – or death – went on.

In the notes sent to the Mortuary, you get a lot of photographs of the patients. When someone has, say, pressure sores or any kind of non-traumatic injury (such as cuts or bad bruises), nursing staff have to take pictures. This is so they can prove that was the condition of the patient on admission and it didn't happen in the hospital. You get all kinds of photographs, especially from a residential home.

If they've been handled, almost inappropriately, certainly quite roughly, you see that when they arrive in hospital. A lot of residential home residents come in with a family unhappy about the care they've received beforehand. They might die in hospital and, while they're happy with all the care they've had in hospital, what they will say is, "Things before weren't too good at all."

There is one residential home in our area where there is a consistent theme of families saying their loved one was left to their own devices. They weren't given drinks, they were left in their room all day and they weren't encouraged to come and engage with anyone else. I'd say over 70 per cent of care home residents who come into hospital and die, have dehydration when they arrive. A lot of them are non-verbal, they have dementia, and it's almost like they're just left. There's that element of it.

You can't take a picture of dehydration, of course, but when you include other things like pressure sores, you do build up a jigsaw puzzle of what's been going on. We often see pictures of necrotic feet and toes, limbs that are absolutely blackened. An image has to be taken when the bandages are removed and sepsis is a really common cause of death. Sepsis has to have come from some source of infection – so, it's a mode of death not a cause of it. You don't naturally develop it. It can be someone who keeps getting UTIs. Or if someone has a pressure sore that no-one has noticed and it gets infected. Or, sometimes, you get people who are just beyond help with it.

When Gerry came into us, his foot was completely black and had been since he'd been taken onto the ward. His family lived quite some distance away and his neighbours used to check up on him and report back. They hadn't seen Gerry for a while, so called his son and daughter. The family asked if the police would go round and they saw that he was stuck when they looked through the letterbox. They called the paramedics and they said as soon as they got access, the smell of decay hit them, and it was all to do with his foot. They took the bandages off and half his foot came with it. He must have been like that for an awfully long time.

Gerry was taken into hospital, where they have sepsis screening as soon as someone is admitted with any infection. Sepsis can develop quite quickly if it isn't cared for properly, particularly in old people. The elderly are susceptible to it as they can suffer from lots of infections. The screening shows whether it is still at the level of an infection or whether it's further and become full-blown sepsis, which can cause all the organs to fail. That can be fatal and can come from something small or from a necrotic foot like Gerry's.

Families are often told their loved one has an infection but, when the cause of death is discussed with them and they're told it was sepsis, they can reel a bit. "Why weren't we told?" is the usual response. It just means that the infection had taken such a hold, and that it quickly developed into the state where it had crossed the line from being a regional infection to flooding the whole body.

Gerry had just said he had "a bad foot" to everyone from paramedics to nursing staff, completely brushing it off. He was still very chatty and resigned to it, apologising for being such a bother because he'd fallen and couldn't get up again with this "bad foot." When we saw the pictures, we couldn't imagine how he had lived with it, there must have been such excruciating pain. It was like something out of a zombie film, dead and coal black. He'd bandaged it up on top of other bandages until those bandages were like papier-mâché, pulpy and green and it must have smelt horrifically.

When the nurses took the bandages off, they had clumps of black flesh stuck to them and his foot was literally down to the bone in certain areas. On the notes, it documented that he was laughing and joking, in good spirits and that he had "no pain." I mean, how can you have no pain when your foot's hanging off? They flooded him with antibiotics – which is how they treat sepsis. If the patient doesn't respond, the treatment is changed to a different type of antibiotics, but there are only so many to try. By that point, sepsis had set in and, ultimately, that's what he died of.

People don't always make the link between something which it looks like the person had been living with well, to then being told they've died of sepsis. They very often feel, "Should we have stepped in sooner? Should something have been done?" Sometimes, you can't stop sepsis developing. It just is what it is, and it will often take a bad path much quicker than is anticipated.

It's really common with pneumonia, as that is an infection that affects your respiratory system and they often go hand-in-hand. It can be so hard for people to hear that is the cause of death. If they know their mum or dad is dying of cancer, then they hear the cause of death is sepsis (because it has to be medically accurate), they don't get what they expected on the certificate. When it's not the words they were expecting, it can be a real shock and I expect many people reading this will have been in that position. It leads them into thinking, *that could have been prevented. We should have done something.* People have the mindset that antibiotics can cure anything, and there is a feeling that death from sepsis could have been avoided.

Going back to Gerry, he was such a frail old man, only about seven stone and in his 80s. He was in a bad way, his skin was breaking down in other parts of his body and he had skin slippage on his arms – yet all of the notes brought across the fact that he was a lovely man. He said that he had no pain, but that couldn't have possibly been the case. It was more likely to just have been the stoical, "Don't bother anyone" attitude that so many old people have. When the antibiotics didn't work, they did discuss amputation of his foot, but he would never have survived the operation. They had a conversation with him to say, "The only way we're going to get rid of this is by amputation." Gerry still had the capacity to make decisions himself and he'd said, "You know what? I'm too old for that. Can you just make me comfortable?" Comfort care was the only other option at that point. They made sure he wasn't in any pain and he died within a few days.

Gerry's family didn't come to view him as they lived so far away but I did speak to them on the phone. They told me he'd had a bad fall. Looking at his foot, that was like saying Fred West was a little bit of a wrong 'un. He'd had a bad foot for years, they said, but looking at those photos, I think it had gone way beyond that description. I don't know how you let something get to that stage, where you are living with something from a horror film on the end of your leg. He'd lived with it so long that it had become his normal, I guess. You get two schools with older people. You get the ones who have the slightest cough and want a drip, or the ones whose leg can be hanging off and they say, "Oh, put a plaster on, it'll be fine." Gerry was one of them.

His daughter said that she'd told him for years to get it looked at, but he wasn't even having district nurses out. Usually, if someone elderly has something like that, they might not be in hospital, but someone in the community will visit to dress it. He had no input from those services at all. No social care involvement, he was just getting on with life himself, on his terms and that was his right. His daughter did ask, "If I'd forced him to get attention, would he have lived?" I don't know. Everyone always wants to know that; if we did this, if we did that, would it have changed things? It might have for a week, a month, but at that stage, with a foot in that condition, he would probably always have died imminently. The fall has just hurried it along a little bit. The slightest little thing would have slipped him over the edge.

We had a lad come in not long after Gerry, who had suffered from mental health problems. He'd had clinical depression for many years, even though he was only 20, and it had worsened. They thought he also had personality disorder but he wouldn't engage with mental health services, so no proper diagnosis could be given. Ross lived with just his dad, after his mum had died – and he spent all his time in his bedroom. His dad would take meals up to him and tried to get Ross out of the bedroom, but he was getting more and more isolated, never leaving the one room towards the end. He spent most of his time gaming and on social media, "happy" in his room. He rarely ate and he never washed or looked after himself. He was brought in because he was unconscious, I'm not sure why. I'd imagine it was a suicide attempt but he also had sepsis.

When you're a parent, you're a parent. It doesn't matter how old your children are, you still have that sense of responsibility and Ross's dad was in bits. Ross was an adult, his dad couldn't have washed him, scrubbed him, or made him have some self-esteem. He had a lot of guilt about the fact that Ross wasn't looking after himself and that he'd known that. He hadn't done anything but could he have done? He'd got mental health services involved but because Ross had capacity and didn't want to engage, you can't force someone. From our perspective – although that doesn't matter – he totally had done everything he could.

You can't take someone kicking and screaming, and force them to change, can you? His jeans were embedded into his skin. He'd urinated in his own clothing and not taken the jeans off for a long time, probably about a year. In the photos, we could see the pattern of the hemp and the lining embedded into his skin when they were removed; his skin just came off with them. It was one of the most extreme things I've ever seen.

When someone like Ross comes in, the hospital will automatically trigger a cause for concern, relating to anyone who is self-neglecting or has any sort of injury or condition which they think could have been prevented. Safeguarding issues had been raised before when Ross had been admitted, and they felt he wasn't able to look after himself. But he'd been assessed and deemed to have capacity. If he wanted to sit in his bedroom and not wash, that was his right. His dad had tried to engage him in things but Ross wasn't having any of it. There are lots of ambiguous causes of death, which cause people to question whether they could have done more, and, of course, there are things they don't understand. Both Ross's dad and Gerry's daughter definitely fell into those categories, and I had no idea how they would move on.

I felt such sadness for Ross, it was such a wasted life. Whereas with Gerry, although that foot might haunt me for years, he'd been cheery and chatty right up to the end. His chattiness couldn't compare to Hetty, though, who came in to see her husband Mick a few days afterwards.

She'd been on the phone a few times and it was hard to get her off the phone. She didn't talk about Mick very much but she was non-stop about everything else.

"I don't know what time I should leave to see him tomorrow, because there are a few roadworks near me and I don't want to be late, if I've told you I'll be there on time. What would you think of me, if I was late? But then again, I don't want to be too early, because then you might think, well, she's a bit disorganised, isn't she? And Mick did always say I was. He would say, 'Oh Hetty, you're that disorganised,' and I'd say, 'You know what, Mick? I am!' So, I'm just wondering, would he tell me to leave early or leave on time? I tell you what I could do, I could leave early, then if I could get through it all OK, I can just pop into Tesco on the way there, pick up a few bits. Mind you, what would I get? I'm just cooking for one now, aren't I? I could always pop any extra in the freezer. But would I remember it was there? Do you know, Mick always used to say I was disorganised?"

Poor woman. I was sure that her stream of consciousness was just covering up her fear that she'd be coming in to see the man she adored, who had dropped dead with no warning the day they came back from visiting their daughter. I didn't need to answer her, she just wanted to go off on one. Hetty must have called about five times the day before she was due to visit Mick and, on her last call that day, after about 20 minutes of non-stop chat about roadworks and Tesco, she asked, "Can I bring any four-legged friends?"

We'd had people asking to bring dogs before. Always dogs, never any other animal. They tended to just leave them with us in the office whilst they viewed, so I passed that information onto Hetty, who then regaled me with tales of various dogs and what they'd got up to over the years.

The next day, she came in, quite bouncy and chipper but, again, I was sure that was hiding her pain. "Still OK for the viewing?" she asked.

"Yes, of course," I replied. "Glad to see the roadworks didn't get in your way!"

"What?" she seemed bewildered by my comment. "Roadworks? Oh, yes, I suppose. I'll just pop back out to the car and get... you know, woof woof! Can you give me a hand?"

I supposed she wanted the dog to see me with her, as I'd be looking after it while she went in to be with Mick. When I got there, she opened up the back of a massive Range Rover and there must have been eight dogs in there! It was like Crufts Central.

"Oh, I'm so sorry," I told her. "There's no way I can let that many dogs into the office."

"The office?" she said. "I want them to come in and see their daddy – say goodbye for one last time."

"Into the viewing area?" I asked, shocked.

"Of course."

"I can't allow that at all, I'd be in breach of pretty much every regulation I can think of."

"And what do you expect me to do? My dogs are very sensitive, you know – simply telling them that Daddy has died won't make them understand. They need to smell him, they need to lick him. They need to see it for themselves."

"Again, I can only apologise, but it just can't happen."

She slammed the door shut and stomped off back to the Mortuary. I asked her if she'd like me to sit with her in the viewing room, to which she sharply replied, "I think not!"

I swear she was in there five minutes or less. Chatty Hetty had turned into the most efficient woman in the world when denied her doggy access. As she left, all I was given was a snorted comment of, "Appalling!" and she disappeared.

Hetty wasn't the only one who, shall we say, "stretched" us. You don't stop having compassion for people but you can be taken aback by some of them! Diana's mum had died from really high blood sugar levels – she was a diabetic and hadn't taken her insulin for some time. She'd died on a Friday night and we didn't receive her body until the Saturday, when we were closed to viewings. I got a call from Diana first thing on the Monday morning.

"You've got my mother," she shouted down the line. "Kathy Hanes! My MOTHER!"

"Yes, we do. I'm so sorry for your loss."

"Don't you start that with me. I know exactly what you're up to. Why wasn't I allowed to see her?"

"I'm really sorry, but we're closed to viewings at weekends. I'd be happy to make an appointment for you now though."

"Oh, I BET you would! Now that you've got what you want!" I was completely in the dark. "I know what goes on at that hospital. I know you take body parts for testing and whatever else you want."

"We don't even perform postmortems here, Diana. This is just somewhere for you to come and say goodbye to your mum if you would like that." I tried to reassure her.

"At the... at the Frankenstein Factory? Everybody knows what you do, everybody knows you keep people away until you've got what you want. Well, let me tell you this... I'm onto you! I'm onto you!" I had a lot of that from Diana over the next few days but she never did come in to see her mother.

While lovely ladies like Diana think we're taking things out, others want us to put things in with their loved ones. It's usually items, such as photographs, teddies or letters but there have been a few stranger ones, too: a stuffed cat (as in taxidermy stuffed, not Bagpuss), a rare comic (that we were told was worth £2000), a Noddy egg cup, some cake and a crash helmet. I think every Mortuary in the country has been asked if the deceased can have a cigarette between their fingers when they go for cremation or burial!

Not to sound heartless, but a lot of losses are very similar. I guess that's the human condition. And just as you think, "This is unusual," there is inevitably something else that comes along to rival it or be even stranger.

We had a death in the community which I found very odd. A young man was brought in by police and we were told there were no suspicious circumstances. Gavin had fallen down the stairs and died but, in the back story somewhere, there was reason to be suspicious, although the police had cleared it.

Wendy said, "This is the one that has allegedly fallen down the stairs."

"Oh, what do you mean 'allegedly'?" I asked. "I thought the police said there were no suspicious circumstances."

"He's got some bruises and scrapes but just wait until you see him."

Gavin was completely intact – except for a massive, cartoon-like wound in his skull, down to his brain on the left-hand side. It was as if someone had just whacked an axe in his head. I found that really hard to let go.

"Come on, let's not be silly here. How can they say that's not suspicious?"

"Well, he's going to the Coroner's Office and the police are investigating, but they don't seem to think there's anything there."

"Wendy. He's been whacked by an axe! Allegedly!"

He did go to the Coroner's Office, as he was deemed to have had an unnatural death by falling, but Gavin really troubled me. If you'd seen his head wound, it was like a prosthetic. He had no marks on him, but the side of his skull was opened up in a straight line as if it had been done precisely with a ruler. Even if he had just fallen, there wouldn't have been a straight line wound like that.

Every time I open a body bag as it's brought in, a new story waits for me. That touches me. When there's a call out, they'll usually ring and say, "Funeral directors are on their way and will meet you there in 15 minutes. It's Margaret Jones for you." They don't say how they died or how old they are. Literally, in that moment when you open the bag, there is a life story lying there.

The first thing to do is unzip the bag so that Margaret's ID can be checked and to make sure it marries up with the information you've been given. But in that moment, as well, you're getting your first glimpse of the person's face. She could have a black tongue or it could be hanging out of her mouth with a ligature still in place – those are all common with hangings. If that's the case, you know what you've got in an instant. Or Margaret might be older, she's got her nightie on and all cleaned up with her fluffy white hair, all ready for bed. Then I know Margaret hasn't had a nasty death, she's probably just passed away in her sleep. Or here's another Margaret who has Valentine's Day pyjamas on and looks as if she could wake up at any moment – I'll probably find out if she's had a heart attack before long. Maybe Margaret has track marks on her arms, or maybe she has blood on her face, or maybe she's a little baby who was named after her great granny but has died in her sleep. I never know until that moment.

I see the face and, if that doesn't tell a story, I see the expression, I see what they're wearing. Sometimes, before I even open the bag, I can smell alcohol or smoke, or a sort of outside smell, if they've been found on the streets or in a park. For me, that has to be the most fascinating moment, as all of life is in that bag of death and I never know what it will be.

I didn't realise that I would learn so much about life through death.

The months I had already spent in this job had changed me forever. The most important thing for me is that I want my family to have resilience once I go – and I was actually seeing that many people achieve that. For the ones who didn't or couldn't, I could see so many points where they could have changed that path. Sometimes, even when someone had clearly been loved – and I've seen this in "real life", too – they could barely even bear to have their name mentioned. I understand that because it can be so painful, but you're not honouring them by doing that. Not only are they not here anymore, they can't even be talked about.

There was one man who was furious when his son walked over to the person in the viewing, and started crying, "Nanna, Nanna!"

"That's enough of that," he said, harshly. "She wouldn't want to see you making a state of yourself."

At no point did he show emotion, at no point did he say "Mum." Who does that help? Not the teenage boy who just wanted to grieve for his nanna while holding her hand, and certainly not the man himself in the long run.

All across the country, people talk in hushed tones about the ones who have died. Mothers and fathers who have lost babies aren't asked their names. People whose partners, spouses or parents are no longer with us are expected, too often, to have a time limit on their grief and then the person will never be mentioned again. The only way to get through grief is to get through it, if that makes sense. The only way to deal with your new normal is to talk about them. You go through the pain barrier that way. It's awful and it's hard, but never having a conversation again about who you've lost is not the way to pay tribute to them.

You can leave houses, you can leave money, you can leave stocks and shares, you can leave jewellery but, ultimately, that will all get diluted as it's passed through the generations. All that can really go on is a memory. You can work every hour of the day and leave it all to your children but, in years to come, when your great-great-great-great grandchildren are around, they won't benefit from that but they might still hear stories about you. Isn't that a better legacy?

If people won't have conversations because they don't want to mention that person, it's almost pointless. When you're young and all the oldies bang on about things, you just want them to shut up. When they go, or when you're that oldie, you would do anything to get an hour with them again. Listen now and make your memories now, because life goes by in a flash and you don't have these chances ever again.

We need to build more emotional resilience. Yes, it's the end of physically being with that person, but you can keep them alive in your own mind, if you have the strength to do so. The love never goes, they still mean the world to you. None of that stops being the case just because they're no longer "here".

They're with you, if you want them to be. They really are.

Chapter 11
March 2020

Around the first week of March, everything changed.

The Mortuary is closed over weekends, so when I turn up on Mondays, there is always a backlog. While we're shut over the weekends, the porters still bring the bodies down. They leave the patient's file on the desk, then we process the paperwork and put it all on the system when we get in on Monday morning.

That first Monday of March, I unlocked the door and saw the pile of red folders. I just thought, *What in the world is going on here?* By March, you'd expect to see the winter numbers really dropping, but this was the opposite. There were so many files that they had been piled on the floor as they would have toppled off the desk. I started to flick through them: *Covid, Covid 19, Covid pneumonia.* The first six I read were all from the same ward.

On the Friday, one of the doctors had spoken to me again about the lung patterns, the cobwebs. "This Covid – we've never seen anything like it before," he'd said.

"I know – you're not the only one telling me that," I'd replied. "Do you think it's going to get as bad as we're hearing?"

He shrugged. "I don't know what's going to happen. It's something completely new to us all. We've no idea how people are contracting this but it won't last long. It'll be over soon."

That Monday was the start of it. This wasn't going to pass in a hurry. Everyone's attitude turned. Those files in front of me, those bodies in the fridges, they were only the ones in our hospital *from* our hospital. They weren't community deaths, they weren't the total from all the hospitals in the area, but they were overwhelming. There can be bad days and bad weekends, but I'd never seen anything as extreme as that. There were dozens of bodies in there, behind the doors, in the fridges. Where would I even begin?

From that day, it was like someone had pressed an alarm button. I'd phone doctors on the wards to try to get them down for the death certificates but no-one was available. People were being admitted faster than they could keep up. There was no-one free for paperwork and they were reticent to come and do it anyway, as they didn't really know what they were dealing with. They knew it was this "Covid thing" but hadn't much of an idea of what that actually was. They saw the news and they saw the X-rays, so they had that. But they were unwilling to acknowledge that it could sweep through populations that quickly.

They were reluctant to complete the cause of death as Covid for these first cases. At the time, to write "Covid" on a death certificate was a really extreme thing to do. It would be an acceptance that it had really hit us. It's so normal now but, back then, it seemed shocking.

I remember the first death certificate that had it as the direct cause. There had been others mentioning it but, in those cases, there had also been a multitude of other things wrong with the patient in question. The death of this man was definitely due to Covid. Technically, he had died of a coronary embolism but, without Covid, he would not have passed. The doctor who came down was trying to find a way to get round what it really was. He, like others, was willing to put it as a contributing factor, if they absolutely had, to but it varied from doctor to doctor.

They couldn't run from it for long because, as that month progressed, the majority of deaths would be from Covid. A team of doctors from pathology and acute medicine came in to complete the death certificates, because there were simply no doctors available. They just stayed there, giving up their own time to complete paperwork. If they hadn't done that, nothing would have moved.

One ward was also allocated as a Covid ward. We were starting to realise just how many mistakes had been made. For too long, patients had been coming in, sitting in

A&E for hours, mingling with everyone and then returning home to spread it further. Or they were taken to a normal ward where the virus could spread and run riot, as medical staff treated the patients without PPE. For so long, it was a free for all, as nothing had been taken seriously. No-one had thought this would amount to anything.

Everything was so quiet and I used some of the time to tidy up the baby room. We have so many donations. People give us clothes and knitwear they no longer need for their babies. Many of them are facing up to the fact that they'll never take their little one home to wear those clothes, but they still think of others.

It was awful to know there were grieving parents out there who were no longer allowed to visit. I'd go to collect the deceased babies from wards and feel the weight of that duty. I'd been doing that for a while. When the porters used the pram to transport the passed babies from the maternity ward, it could lead to an awkward situation. It's such an old-fashioned pram – and the natural reaction is for people to try to see the baby. It was so unusual and old fashioned, that people would say, "Let's have a look!"

You'd have to carry on walking quickly. It does have a big square hood with a little lip, and we would put a fabric mesh on it and just say, "Sorry, have to go!" It was more natural to see a woman pushing it than a porter. It was meant to be a gentler, more natural way of transporting the babies but it wasn't without problems. No-one ever looked in fully, but there was always that worry, so we stopped doing it. With Covid raging, though, there was no chance of that happening now, as there was no-one wandering about.

The ladies who knit items for us, do clothing for all sizes. They had now started making love hearts. They made them in sets of two – we put one in the baby's hand and gave one to the mum. There are little silver angels from SANDS that work that way too, one for baby, one for mum. I always wondered what stories those ladies had.

By the time measures such as masks and gowns, specific wards and social distancing were implemented, Covid had taken a real hold on things. It was across the country, not just in our area. Within a few weeks, we knew we were in trouble. We barely had time to look up, it was constant. Usually, we would have some lighter moments – not now. The hospital began isolating the Covid wards and that changed everything. We couldn't let anyone into the Mortuary for viewings. All of those bereaved people suddenly had nowhere to go and their grief was in limbo. The very heart of what we did was stopped.

Our instructions were basic: *Don't let anyone in; this is highly contagious.* There was no humanity to that but, as we'd been told many times by doctors, *we're here for the living, not the dead.* The thing was, down in the Mortuary, we were there for both.

The very thought of people not being able to see their loved ones hit me hard. I always, always, treated the bodies with respect and dignity but I now felt even more commitment to that. Those of us who worked in the Mortuary would be the only visitors now. For months, I had been hearing those phrases from families: *Will she be lonely? I don't like to think of him here by himself.* Now I knew what they meant. It wasn't a silly thought (not that I'd ever felt that way), there really was a sense of being alone.

I remember the last viewing, before the rules changed, very clearly. We've obviously had lots of same sex couples but because Mark was the last grieving visitor allowed into the Mortuary to see his loved one, this couple seemed very special to me. Mark and Ronnie had only got married five years ago, but had been together for 40 years all in. They were both in their 70s but Mark had been married, and had had kids, before he and Ronnie had finally found their way to be together.

Mark was utterly broken by his loss. "Is it OK to just sit here and talk to him for a bit?" he asked me.

"Take as long as you like," I replied. "Do you want me to leave you with your husband?"

"No, no. You can stay, that's fine."

"I know it's hard, I know it's so hard."

"Oh well, we had it hard for a long time. We were shunned you know. No-one wanted to even look at us, speak to us, they couldn't bear to be anywhere near us. Back then…" his voice trailed off. "Do you remember?" he said to Ronnie. "The world's changed now, and thank goodness for that but, back then, we never knew whether we were even going to get home in one piece if we went out together. The words people said to us, the beatings we got… but I was lucky. I got to have him."

It sounded like Mark had been through an awful time, for so long, as people wouldn't accept his sexuality. But all he was talking about was the fact that things had changed, and he was so lucky to have this man in his life.

"Do you have any support Mark?" I asked.

"Oh yes, I've got four children and they're all there for me now. I married very young, it was just the done thing to do. They accepted who I was eventually. Eventually." He emphasised that word, and I could only imagine what his life had been like. "They're worried about me now, but they needn't be. I'll be OK. I've had this wonderful man in my life for 40 years and it was all worth it."

And that was it. Mark was my last visitor.

The mortality numbers were rising thick and fast, and the common theme was Covid coating the lungs. Doctors could identify that clear pattern and they now knew it was exactly the virus they'd been warned about.

Before long, ICU was full, there were no beds left and wards were changing by the day. When we went into lockdown, full PPE was being used across the whole hospital, as well as face masks being introduced. The acute medicine ward got changed to a ward just for Covid. But this meant I didn't know how to get hold of doctors, or which wards were now Covid central. If someone tested positive, it was easier to make it a Covid ward than get infection control in to clean everything, because by the time they came in, another case had been found. It was utter chaos.

We had to fight things on two fronts – not only were we dealing with numbers unlike anything we'd faced before, but we couldn't have people coming into the hospital any more as we went into lockdown.

I think I approach death and dying in quite a pragmatic way. I do what I can for the people we care for, both those who have gone and those who are left behind. But I'm struggling with these next sentences. During Covid, people couldn't say goodbye to their loved ones. They just weren't allowed. Nurses were helping them to video call on mobile phones and tablets. It was something none of us, no-one in the world, could ever have imagined. There were people at the very end of life who never knew that final hug or final kiss from their husband, wife or partner, their child or their parent.

One of the most upsetting things were the Covid patients who had gone in, completely aware and lucid. They weren't collapsing and there were no dramatics. They were unwell with this virus. For them to be told, *The only way we can resolve this is by intubating you and, if we intubate you, there is a very high chance you won't wake up again*, is the stuff of nightmares.

These were ordinary people who were poorly but they had often been at work the week before. There was no slow decline, it had just hit them like a ton of bricks. They were actually having to make a decision which could kill them, just in the hope that they might be one of the few who were saved. They were agreeing to intubation because they couldn't breathe – what choice is that? Facetiming their families, their spouses, their children, saying, *I've decided to be intubated; if I don't wake up, I love you.* Making those calls must have taken more strength than I can even imagine – receiving them would haunt you for the rest of your days. They'd be giving the thumbs up before they closed the screen. It was beyond heart-breaking and the impact on staff must have been huge, too.

At the start, when someone died up in ICU, the staff were wrapping the notes up and isolating them for 48 hours. I don't even know where that idea had come from but how were we going to effectively manage the whole post-death process if we had that sort of delay? Deaths were still meant to be registered within five days, no rules had changed. If we weren't given access to the notes for 48 hours, we'd lost two full days. People were just guessing about so much. There were no hard and fast rules. Staff didn't know enough about Covid to know whether the virus was still on the notes and active after 48 hours. It was all very good wrapping it all up in sheets or bags, but we still had to touch it all. It was crazy and just one indication of how desperate everyone was to contain this virus that was sweeping through everywhere.

Towards the end of March, we ran out of body bags and people had to be wrapped in sheets. Supplies were low in every Mortuary in the country, so it wasn't a matter of just ordering them from somewhere else. It seemed as if everything was falling to pieces. Even the way in which bodies were brought to us was different now. Previously, when someone died out of hours, the porters would bring them to the Mortuary. A risk assessment had determined they shouldn't be doing that now. They were instructed not to handle the bodies which meant they couldn't even go onto the wards. The bodies were wheeled to them, already prepared at the door of the ward.

This meant that we were getting constant out-of-hours callouts, too. It was still just a team of three – me, Wendy and Gary – and there was always one of us on call. Every time there was a Covid death during the week between 6pm and 9am, or over the weekend, whoever was on duty would have to go to the Mortuary and then to the ward to get the body.

The porters used a concealment trolley and brought them to the Mortuary but they weren't allowed to handle the bodies and put them in the fridges. They weren't allowed contact at all. They'd get a call to say someone had died on a Covid ward, then they would ring the on-call Mortuary technician.

"We've got a Covid one coming in at 4am," we'd be told. "Meet you there."

I'd roll out of bed, usually deciding it would be best to just keep my pyjamas on and throw a coat over the top, and drive to the Mortuary. I'd get my PPE on, sort out the fridge and wait for the porter to come. Before Covid, they would usually help you, but it wasn't an option now. There would be a cursory handing over, both parties scared to infect the other, then I would be left alone with the trolley and the deceased. It was a real struggle. At the start, there were so many people dying who were overweight and it was tough for me to get a bigger body into the fridge space, which was becoming full by now. We just had to cope.

There were times when I had less than an hour of sleep a night. We were dead on our feet – just like everyone else in the morgue! We used to do a week at a time on call. We were still doing day shifts, too, but now we had to do it night-by-night. Getting called out was relentless. You could be there at 2am for one, and while waiting there would be another call to say someone else was coming, or you'd put the body away and be in the car to go home when a call would say another one was on the way. With just the three staff, it was hard to think we could maintain this way of life. All the doctors were banging on about herd immunity and we thought, we just needed to hang on for a bit and things would get under control.

Masks and PPE were the be-all and end-all. Even at stupid o'clock, in the dark, alone and with no idea if it could even be transmitted by a corpse, we all wore masks. They were dark days – and nights – only made bearable by the team spirit and dedication that we all shared.

At one point, someone kept leaving flowers and candles in the Mortuary car park. There were no names on the containers, so no-one could have known who was in them unless they worked there. We never saw anyone delivering them but, in the same spot, under a tarpaulin, there were several small bouquets and some tealight candles that had been lit as the person left. We never did find out who it was, but I think maybe people were finding other ways to say goodbye.

We still thought it would be temporary, we still thought we'd be through it soon. The tealights would stop, the viewings would start, we'd look back on these weeks, and think, *Well, that was weird.* We knew nothing.

Chapter 12
April 2020

The relentless way of existing caused by Covid continued into April. We just felt our way, there was no map to guide us. It was all so unexpected, which seems naïve given the warnings, but things hadn't come true with other viruses, and this had happened almost out of the blue. I tested positive for antibodies and lots of people who had been ill at Xmas did, too. It had definitely been around for a good few months, before anyone really knew what it was. The Trust claimed that eight per cent of staff in the hospital had either had Covid in the past or were currently dealing with it, but the rate amongst the five of us in the Mortuary was 100 per cent. Something didn't add up.

Obviously, we were still in isolation in April, with the three of us working until we were fit to drop. Cases were piling up, with harrowing stories coming from all sides. The world was in lockdown but ours wasn't exactly a job you could do from home.

Staff in a big hospital are always busy and under pressure, but they were in tears all the time. There were people who were too scared to come into work, as they feared they'd give it to their kids, others who just wanted to lock themselves away. Everybody was terrified, it was bordering on hysteria. So many doctors were off poorly, they'd tested positive, and we couldn't get replacement staff. Everything had a knock-on effect, and the level of care people were getting had to be compromised, as there just weren't the staff to do it all.

"Normal" deaths were still going on but families couldn't come in for viewings – and I have to admit that affected me. I'd been in this job for quite a while now, I'd found my way, and I got satisfaction from helping people navigate death. That had all been thrown up in the air – none of us knew what was happening and our routes through the final stages of life had never been so unpredictable.

When it was a Covid death, it almost validated the fact that we couldn't allow visitors in. However, when someone had died on a non-Covid ward of a non-Covid death – which was becoming quite rare – families couldn't really accept why we wouldn't allow them to see their loved one. We had to trot out, "It's the Trust policy now, we have to follow national guidelines." There were no exceptions. People turned up at the door, saying, "I want to see my mum, please let me see her," or "I want to kiss my dad one last time," and we had to be hard line. It was awful.

An added problem was that some nurses hadn't considered that the lockdown applied to the Mortuary.

People turning up didn't always know they'd get knocked back – sometimes a person would ask if they could see their deceased loved one, and a nurse would say, "I'm sure the Bereavement Office will sort it out. Go and contact them." They would turn up the next day, and we'd be there with the bad news. "What do you mean I can't? They wouldn't let me into the ward – they said I could come and see him here. Are you going to stop me saying goodbye? Are you actually going to stand there and say I can't?" There was hysteria – and I understood it. You felt like you were playing, God.

I lost count of the number of times I had to say, "No, you can't see your loved one, I'm incredibly sorry."

"But he hasn't died of Covid," I'd be told.

It didn't matter.

It was horrible, I just felt like I wanted to get away. I wanted to do good and lighten the load for everyone, as they were all at breaking point, It was hard to see how long we could maintain it, every aspect of Covid was already relentless. The administration was relentless, the emotional drain was relentless, even having conversations with doctors who were in tears was relentless. Every aspect was so draining. That's something I found really hard – it was all out of our hands. I would have lost my job if I'd given a viewing.

For a few baby deaths, I did ask.

"If the building is empty? If everyone is in full PPE? If it's only 10 minutes? Can we please allow a viewing?"

There was never any bending at all. It was always knocked back. That information didn't filter round to all ward staff or they just didn't realise it meant the Mortuary, too. Having bereaved parents turn up in floods of tears will haunt me forever.

People will never get over these things. We put up a plaque for all who died in the hospital already. It said: *You weren't able to hold them, you weren't able to take them home, but they were looked after and cared for here.* It was purely a recognition that it had happened. No-one came to see it then, I don't know if they ever will. People didn't want to return, as they felt they had been cheated. Also, during those early days, I think there was a feeling that it would happen to someone else. But for those who came in for routine operations and developed Covid, that was different. Families would say, "I kept them safe at home since this pandemic started, they came into hospital and they got it and died."

What do you say to that? I felt I was ruining lives and, for the first time, I was bone-tired. Not saying goodbye, not seeing loved ones in person, video calling people before they died, it affected everyone. We weren't allowed to do video calls in the Mortuary which was odd – it had been something I had hated when I caught people doing it and, yet, now we could all see that it might have some value. It felt like a plague, like we were in some surreal futuristic hell. Every day we all wondered, is this really happening? It was almost as if the world was ending, an apocalypse was coming, and things had changed in an instant. There was a feeling in the hospital and Mortuary, where we were at the centre of it, *If this can change so dramatically, what will happen next?*

In April, it was just appalling. One night, just before a change in staff, I was leaving at 10pm (much later than pre-Covid) when it all seemed so overwhelming. The pathology doctors had been in doing paperwork for us all day but we were still so behind. Ward doctors didn't have to see the body after death, as any unnecessary exposure was trying to be restricted. So, we couldn't stick to the previous rule of having to involve a doctor who had seen the patient alive. We had to muddle through, though, and these wonderful pathology doctors had been helping out since the start.

The pathology doctors were coming on their days off, when they had a free hour, all the time. Then they'd go home to their families, with no idea whether they were carrying the virus with them. I was coming in at 7am, going home at 10pm – we all did that. If we'd had a day when we couldn't get paperwork done, we wouldn't have coped. We were like the walking dead.

We had gowns that went on frontways, gloves, masks and headgear – and we had to wear all of that, all the time. I don't think I was scared at that point because I thought I'd definitely had Covid at Xmas, and there had been lots of staff off at that point with the same symptoms, especially the distinctive one of losing the sense of smell. I was so focused on having so much to do. April was the height of it so far, and we consistently saw about 12 cases a night every night. Then on a Monday, after the weekend, there would be at least 40 cases when we came in. The doctors who weren't involved in the care of a patient, didn't know what that patient was like. They were just being parachuted into whatever case, whatever ward needed them at that moment.

If there was a positive Covid test in the notes, that meant it was counted as a Covid death. If they hadn't done that, if they hadn't just gone for a shortcut at times, I don't know what we would have done. A lot of those deaths were probably primarily down to something else but it was so overwhelming. If Covid was there in the notes, it was Covid. Head accident? He tested positive, so it was Covid. Car crash? She tested positive, so it was Covid. It wasn't out of malpractice, it was purely the workload. If the doctors hadn't done that, people would never have had their loved ones released. It wasn't ideal but, even now, I don't know what the answer would have been.

In April, I felt we'd never get back to what we'd had before. Everyone was so down, no-one had anything to look forward to: we weren't seeing anyone or going anywhere, and we were dealing with this plague on a daily basis. Fear was everywhere. There was no vaccination, there were nightly press conferences and people were talking about herd immunity. You queued to get into the supermarket, with health workers wearing passes so they could get back to work as quickly as possible, or to do their shopping quickly after an 18-hour shift.

We clapped on the doorsteps for the NHS, went one way round the shops, washed our shopping and didn't even go for a walk, unless it was beside our house. It had all happened so quickly, yet we had no choice but to accept everything. So many doctors left. They just couldn't deal with the workload or the expectations. One of our best consultants was in ICU and nearly died. He was so bad that his wife was brought in to say goodbye to him. When we heard that he had pulled through, my first thought was, *How will that poor man ever deal with coming back to the Mortuary, realising he could have been one of the statistics here?*

When you drove onto the hospital grounds, it was eerie. There were no signs of people walking together or chatting as they went for lunch. There was no camaraderie – just tumbleweed.

One day, I needed to go onto a ward to ask a doctor a question. I called up and was told, "There's no way he can leave. You'll have to come here and we'll give you full PPE." I wasn't prepared for the scene which hit me when I walked into that ward. It was like a dystopian film. All of the doctors were wearing welding mask-type face coverings, full hoods, boots and huge gloves. There was a moment when I looked around, saw them all dressed like that and heard the noises of everyone who couldn't breathe – ventilators for some, hideous rasping breaths for others – and it was gruesome. I looked and saw it from the patient's perspective: people who were there to care for them were dressed up like astronauts and the noises that were coming from the beds were unreal. People were being wheeled out dead, and there was no chance for even a moment of normality. It was surreal – what the hell had the world come to?

Covid made us all face death in such an unpredictable way. Our own mortality, and that of our loved ones, was compounded by the scale of loss which played out on our TV screens every night for months. Behind every number was a life. I suppose it made people face death in a way we did in the Mortuary every day – but in such an intense way. People were coming into hospital for conditions and operations which had made them very poorly, not routine appointments, but situations which needed treatment as soon as possible. However, they were being told that they were basically doing it at their own risk. "We appreciate you need this treatment but the chances are, if you come into hospital, you might end up with Covid and you might die," were the words used. They had to make an informed decision as to whether it was worth it – but was it truly informed? The level of care couldn't be guaranteed, there was backlog quickly growing, and we never knew which staff levels would be provided. Not everyone who died that month died *from* Covid, but Covid had still got them in a sense.

I'd never been so shattered in my life and everyone around me felt the same way. If we'd known, *you have to do this for another two weeks,* or *just one more month,* it would have given light at the end of the tunnel. There was nothing like this. It was the new normal. One night, when I was playing

Jenga with the bodies, I felt a tear in my abdomen. It was a hiatus hernia but I had to keep going. Unless you had Covid, unless you needed to isolate, you couldn't stop.

We were chosen to receive what is called a National Asset. It is basically a plan and infrastructure for mass casualties, and it is put in place if there needs to be a response to something which causes more than the usual number of deaths. For us, that meant that we got a building that could hold 250 bodies and "Nutwells". Nutwells are temporary body storage units – we were crying out for something, as there was virtually no space left in the Mortuary. The fridges were almost full.

When someone is booked in, their measurements are booked in, too. That's one of the first things a funeral director will ask for, when they call. You'll say, "I've got Joan, she's 5' 3" and 18" across." This always happens but, with the Nutwells, it became even more important. Whereas Mortuary fridges are metal trays that come out so that the bodies can slide onto them, Nutwells are almost like a very shallow bath, slidable scoops really. They're acrylic and where you would have a handle in a bath, they have a strap which is what you use to pull and move them. The sides are curved and sloped, so the surface area is reduced – this means that the deceased has to be small, less than 16" across. Not many people are when their arms are crossed, so there were few that would fit without being manhandled. We had to go through the bodies and identify the ones that would fit in the Nutwells.

After joiners built the shell of a new building in the parking area, these temporary Nutwells were put in place. We had sixty of them and while it was good to have extra spaces, they were tiny. The Mortuary itself could hold 120, and the National Asset could hold 250. The National Asset was never used and I have no idea why not. If it had been, we could have avoided the appalling situation we ended up in. Towards the end of April, we had a situation where all the "normal" slots were full as well as some Nutwells, but no-one was arriving who was small enough to use any more of those.

I don't know how, maybe it was luck, but everything did keep moving, even though we were pretty much at capacity, sometimes even down to just one space. We had to move bodies about and it was hard. On top of that, was the frustration that this all-singing, all-dancing National Asset was just sitting there, not being used. We were always on the brink: *If we have a busy night, what will we do?* was the question on our minds. We were constantly trying to get people moving.

Even the funeral directors didn't want to touch Covid bodies or have them in the chapels of rest. They wouldn't allow families to drop things off for them, and they tried to seal everything off from Covid, if they could. Everything was so new and alien. Nobody wanted to be around us. The Mortuary was viewed as if it was the hub of Covid – maybe it was symbolic, as we were the centre of death at the best of times, anyway. Yet, the reality was, these people had died on the wards! They hadn't died with us but we were being shunned. We were doing all we could to protect ourselves but people were so reticent about coming anywhere near us. They seemed to think of us as Covid central but there was never any evidence to suggest that the virus was still active once someone died. It was airborne and travelled through the respiratory system, so if someone wasn't breathing, it shouldn't be there. It seemed obvious.

Funerals weren't taking place and we saw a huge increase in direct cremations. They had happened every so often in the past, but Covid really made those take off. Rather than only have two people at a cremation, families were opting to have the body taken directly from us, cremated, and then just be given the ashes at a later date. When people started talking about the numbers getting uncontrollable, some funeral directors even raised the possibility that we might need to look at mass cremations. How had we got here?

So many of the actions and so much of the dialogue around Covid was almost medieval. The body was seen as an infected source, that few people understood – and we had the biggest cross of all on our door. We were holding death, even if we weren't creating it. It really was the time of the plague.

We're not too good at dealing with death in this country, anyway, and this was now being reinforced. It was as if someone bigger than us was saying: *Here is this huge thing happening that we don't know how to deal with at the best of times— and now it's just going to be shoved into your lives without any choice. You don't know who will get it or who will die. Good luck!*

People who would never have normally had a conversation about death were forced to confront it. There were some who folded but, as always, good people showed they were good people. The camaraderie between us as a team and other departments was amazing. We were all under so much pressure but there was support and everyone did what they could. If there was anything positive, it was that everyone was just that little bit more forgiving as everyone was scared. *Next week, it could be me or someone I love.* Everyone knew that we were all going through something horrible, so if someone was narky one day, that was fine. We were all under pressure and things could slide until the situation got better or we were stronger.

We had to be family for each other. The Mortuary team always was the underdog of the hospital but it was even more so now. It was so challenging and awful but, I think, the impact it had on people was that it made them that little more forgiving and that was a silver lining. We got through it because of each other. I never minded going to work during those months, in fact, it was another home because of the people I was with. I suppose, before Covid, I had an almost pastoral care role and that was taken away from me. I missed it massively. I just wasn't dealing with families doing viewings any more. I had my hands tied, we all did. The essence of what we once did, the tangible stuff, the viewings, the sitting down with people for hours on end and letting them talk and show photos, all stopped. The buzzer never went. No-one came. We all struggled with the change of working practices but also with the feeling that we were letting people down. We knew what was going on outside of our walls and there was nothing we could do.

People and babies didn't stop dying of other things. In particular, there was such an influx of suicides because of the impact on mental health. It became heartbreakingly obvious. At one point, we had five young people at once who had all taken their lives in one way or another. People didn't have their outlets of gym or friends. There was nothing. There was a price paid for that and we were seeing it so horribly clearly.

I think, with some people, there was still a bit of denial – the elderly who died, would have probably died of any virus. If you have pre-existing conditions, you're always more at risk. However, I still couldn't believe that, only a month before, we thought we'd only see a few cases: people who were already frail and unwell, and that would be the extent of this "Covid". We went up to eight wards designated just for the virus. The volume of patients grew and the staff levels reduced as one by one, doctors, nurses and various staff became ill, or showed symptoms and had to take time off. People dying in care homes were brought in, too – it was spreading so quickly in those places.

Apart from ambulances, the hospital grounds were empty. Our disposable boilersuits and sealed wellies with facemasks and gloves made everything feel so claustrophobic. It seemed as if Covid was the only topic on the agenda, whether that be on the news or at work – but people still continued to die of other things too. Their families still grieved for them and had to go through the same pain, but with the added distress of not being allowed to see them or say goodbye. This was tough enough when it was largely the elderly, but Covid didn't discriminate and soon it affected people of all ages.

Previously healthy people who had come in for routine procedures, contracted Covid and died very quickly. Their families endured a sudden, wrenching loss. There was no way of preparing or saying goodbye, or even understanding what this virus was that had taken someone they loved, so quickly and cruelly. The pain in their voices was indescribable when, time and time again, we had to tell them that they wouldn't be able to see their loved one for one final time. Hardened doctors and nurses were in tears, as they described having to tell the families of young people, just starting out in life, that they weren't going to be coming home and the only way to say goodbye was via a screen on their phone. It was surreal and devastating, and we all existed in a state of sleep-deprived sadness, that was unrelenting, for what seemed like forever.

We had to keep the Covid deaths separate or contained together in one strip. If we'd had, for example, three long termers taking up one whole row of fridges, that would have caused problems as we'd have had to turn bodies away.

"Have you ever run out of space?" I asked Wendy. "What if that happens? I know we're close but what will we actually do if it does occur?"

"It has happened before, actually," she replied. "There was one awful winter, maybe ten years ago, and everything came to a standstill because of the level of snow we had. I had to put mattresses on the floor of the postmortem room and wrap bodies in sheets. All the other hospitals were full as well and we couldn't move the bodies on. I just couldn't leave someone lying on the floor – they needed dignity, didn't they? We must have been about ten over at that time. If we have to do it again, we will. We'll just have to."

Did it all affect me? Absolutely. More so than anything of the previous months. Will I carry it into the rest of my life? Without a doubt. None of us will be immune from that, will we? I think everyone has had a glimpse of how life can change in an instant, not just from someone dying, but from the world altering with hardly any notice. A combination of seeing the wreckage from Covid and working with the dead flicked a switch in me, to the point where I was writing letters in my head to my children, as I was terrifyingly worried about how they would cope without me. Even although they're all in their late teens and 20s, you never stop needing your mum, do you? The thought obsessed me. I wouldn't be there to comfort them, they would have to go through every single thing in their lives without me if I died now, and it was just too soon. I didn't have a fear of death before, in fact, I was a very easy-going person without any anxiety. Now, I would say, although I still don't fear death at all – it's inevitable and we can all guarantee it'll happen – it has started to feel more imminent. I'm 50 now and the clock's ticking.

I think that before I dealt with death all the time, there wasn't such a sense of time running out. I think about it constantly now, and that's what I don't like. None of us knows how long we've got with our families and every moment seems precious.

I don't worry about me dying because I think when you're gone, you're gone. It's about worrying things are too late for me. It's not even a fear of death, as I just won't be here any more. But I do have this constant worry that time is running out and I don't want people being left behind, at a time that isn't right. That is the focus. If I had got poorly and terminally ill, before the Mortuary and before Covid, I would have been OK about it. Now, I stub my toe and think I'll get sepsis, and be dead in a week! It's not about being scared, it's about seeing how quickly it all goes, how unpredictable it all is and how much I want my kids settled before I leave. Seeing women younger than me in the Mortuary is strange, because the effect has been to completely desensitise me to the act of dying. Being gone is fine. I just want the opportunity to experience all the things in life I can, and for the kids to be in a place where they are able to handle it, at a time when it is more expected.

The way we approach death can make life all the more precious. Everyone has lost someone dear, everyone has questions about this stage of our common experience, but nothing had prepared me for what I'd gone through. For a year, I'd been dealing with death in the middle of death, and yet Covid was something that came as a bolt from the blue rather than "normal" death and it affected me in a way I could never have predicted. The elderly, the ill, those who choose to take their own lives – all of that was miles away from seeing previously healthy young and middle-aged people arrive in the Mortuary, after only a few days of ill health with this virus we had all dismissed.

Covid hadn't changed the basics of death – whoever was grieving still felt pain, loss, sadness, exhaustion, love and emptiness. They were just feeling it in a world that now had no anchor. We rely on science to help us delay and avoid death – and now it wasn't working fast enough. Science is there to help when our loved ones have cancer or tumours, when a baby is born too early, or a child is brought in from an accident almost too late. It is there with needles and vials and operating tables and anaesthetics. It is there to save lives and prolong them. What do we do when science is being outrun by a virus that we can't see but which is after us all?

The death of someone who has a terminal illness or is very old may not come as a surprise, but it is still a shock. Now, we were all being shocked every day. Young people were dying, healthy people were dying, our elderly were locked away from us and we couldn't be there in their final days. People said goodbye through care home windows, if they were lucky, others died after having seen no-one but staff for weeks on end. I truly believe it will take many, many years for us all to come back from that, if we ever do. Covid changed life, and it changed death.

If we have loved them, we can carry the dead with us if we choose to do so. This isn't a religious approach, it's just something which can bring some comfort. We all need that.

Death is our biggest enemy – no wonder we fight it, and no wonder we deny it as much as we can. It will always win, and we know that. For so many of us, the process of death is hidden, in nursing homes, hospitals and hospices where someone else takes care of it. It used to happen at home, where the elderly or the terminal would be cared for by their families. Of course, in past times when medicine and outside help were luxuries for the rich, there weren't always options, but death wasn't hidden away so much. Now, we expect quantity over quality of life, but it's often someone else providing everything which will facilitate that. We just don't see death any more. And that makes us terrified.

We're all mortal, we can't outrun it; but maybe we could embrace it just a little more, knowing it will come for us one day and try to live life to the full before that day arrives. That doesn't negate or minimise heartache – the mother who loses a baby suffers an agony that should never happen. It's different with children, it's different for those who die too young but, for those who are blessed with a life that covers many decades, if they can just think *There is still life to be had*. No matter how small the terms of that life may have become, maybe there can be something there.

It's hard, isn't it? I'm not trying to say death and dying are something to celebrate but life is, and both are inextricably linked. We just can't consider a good death without a good life.

What medicine can hide, death reveals. Once a life is over, a viewing opens it all up again. Looking at the body of a person you love can expose so much that was hidden by their time in hospital or in a hospice. The bare truth lies in the viewing room. Mystery and death exist side-by-side behind the doors of the Mortuary, and I hope that by taking you on a journey beyond, I've tackled that mystery a little bit. Death ensures that we lose control but we can take a little control back, by understanding what goes on before it happens and that grief throws us into a world of unknowns.

As Elisabeth Kubler-Ross said: "Dying is an integral part of life, as natural and predictable as being born. But whereas birth is a cause for celebration, death has become a dreaded and unspeakable issue to be avoided by every means possible in our society... we may be able to delay it, but we cannot escape it... And death strikes indiscriminately, it cares not at all for the status or position of the ones it chooses; everyone must die, whether rich or poor, famous or unknown. Even good deeds will not exclude their doers from the sentence of death; the good die as often as the bad. It is perhaps this inevitable and unpredictable quality that makes death so frightening to many people. Especially those who put a high value on being in control of their own existence are offended by the thought that they, too, are subject to the forces of death."

No way of grieving is right and no way of grieving is wrong – but with each loss, I feel that we should take a moment to linger, to sit in that loss and ask, *What now?* It's a time to reflect on whether our own life is at a crossroads, whether the lost one was someone dear, or just an acquaintance. It gives us a chance to pause and wonder how our next moments, days, months and years will be lived, because no-one knows when it will be their moment to leave.

After all, death doesn't define us – life does.

Goodbye

The clock is always ticking, the sand is always falling – we can't do anything about that.

But there is always hope and there is always love.

We only have now and there's absolutely no point dwelling on what happened yesterday, and none of us know if we'll even be sitting here this time tomorrow.

As I write this, I'm waiting on my first grandchild coming. I'll love him to bits, I'll tell him stories and teach him as much as I can. He'll be adored and with a bit of luck, one day – years and years from now hopefully – he'll be telling his own children about me.

I've lived among the dead for longer than I would have thought, and they have taught me more than I could ever have imagined. I think I've found my place here, I think I feel like I belong. I'm not ready to join them yet but, if I could reach out and thank each and every one of them for adding to the tapestry that has brought me to this place of understanding, I would.

Sorry for your Loss

How can I end something that will never end? We'll all go through this and all that I know is that love will be what matters when it's your time. Don't be afraid to show affection, don't be afraid to stop working and listen to old stories, don't be afraid of what lies behind the curtain.

You'll be fine and someone, somewhere will be genuinely sorry for your loss. x

Acknowledgements

I'd like to thank my work family for making the worst of times, the best of times – particularly, Wednesday Adams (love you), Foxy, and Scoff.

Huge thanks to everyone who consented to their experiences being included in this book and to all the amazing and dedicated healthcare professionals that I have met along the way (there are too many of you to list, but I appreciate every single one of you).

To my real-life family for continuing to support and believe in me.

To the team at Mardle, particularly Jo Sollis for making this book possible.

To ghostwriter Linda Watson-Brown – you continue to inspire me, make me laugh and feel a little less crazy. I might have to put you in the friend category at this rate!

Thank you for all your continued support, advice and wisdom.

A very special lady once said to me: *Nothing ever ends, not really.* She was right. My children will continue to feel my love long after I'm gone, just as we still feel hers. We love you, Mamma, and we miss you every day.